ONE MEDICINE

ONE MEDICINE

HOW UNDERSTANDING ANIMALS
CAN SAVE YOUR LIFE

DR MATT MORGAN

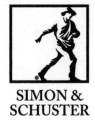

**SIMON &
SCHUSTER**

London · New York · Sydney · Toronto · New Delhi

First published in Great Britain by Simon & Schuster UK Ltd, 2023

Copyright © Matt Morgan, 2023

The right of Matt Morgan to be identified as the author of this work has been
asserted in accordance with the Copyright, Designs and Patents Act, 1988.

1 3 5 7 9 10 8 6 4 2

Simon & Schuster UK Ltd
1st Floor
222 Gray's Inn Road
London WC1X 8HB

www.simonandschuster.co.uk
www.simonandschuster.com.au
www.simonandschuster.co.in

Simon & Schuster Australia, Sydney
Simon & Schuster India, New Delhi

The author and publishers have made all reasonable efforts to contact
copyright-holders for permission, and apologise for any omissions or errors in the form
of credits given. Corrections may be made to future printings.

A CIP catalogue record for this book is available from the British Library

Hardback ISBN: 978-1-4711-7307-3
Trade Paperback ISBN: 978-1-4711-7308-0
eBook ISBN: 978-1-4711-7309-7

Typeset in Bembo by M Rules
Printed and Bound in the UK using 100% Renewable Electricity
at CPI Group (UK) Ltd

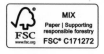

MIX
Paper | Supporting
responsible forestry
FSC® C171272
FSC
www.fsc.org

To my three beautiful girls Alison, Evie and Mimi.
I love you to the moon and back.

'Some people talk to animals. Not many listen though. That's the problem.'

A. A. Milne, *Winnie-the-Pooh*

Contents

Author's Note

I have changed some of the personal details of patients to help protect their privacy. Where cases are likely to disclose a patient's identity through their unusual nature, I have sought patient consent — or assent from their relatives — to share these details with the reader. While all clinical cases are based on real patients, some names and characteristics may have been changed, some events compressed and some dialogue recreated. I have only included facts that I believe to be true, although I have not sought independent verification of second-hand details given to me by colleagues, families or friends.

Introduction

It all started when Barry choked on a Hobnob. He suffered a cardiac arrest after the oat biscuit went into his lungs instead of his stomach and ended up in my intensive care unit. I nearly came to a similar fate that same morning. It was a rare hot Welsh summer day and I had inhaled countless flies during my bike ride along the river to work. Had I ridden into a bee, I too may have been battling for my life.

As we tried to save Barry's life, a flock of birds flew past the hospital window next to his bed. Why don't those birds die? I thought. Although not known for their love of biscuits, birds continually inhale things that could block their lungs as they fly forwards. How do they survive? I wondered. And so, my obsession with what animals can teach us about human medicine was born – from a simple Hobnob.

Barry survived and so did my enthusiasm for the subject. Then the questions really started. Every day in intensive care, I meet people at the brink of life. When I try to understand their disease and think of treatments, I now see animals. How does a giraffe breathe and can it help us treat asthma? Why do kangaroos have three vaginas and can it help couples having IVF? Why do koalas eat shit and should I feed it to my own children? How can an ant help stop the pandemic? Is this strange? Yes, I suppose so. But using solutions nature invented millions of years ago to solve twenty-first-century problems shouldn't be that strange.

And so began my quest. Along the way, I would uncover an age-old relationship between humans and animals. It would take me to places far away and places under my nose that I never knew existed. My journey would be rudely interrupted by a viral pandemic that would underline how human and animal medicine can, and must, be brought closer together. Made one. One Medicine.

Where better to start this journey than with the original fusion between human and animal – the work of Charles Darwin. His pioneering journey on HMS *Beagle* rocked the worlds of medicine, of science and of life itself. With my tickets booked, my bags packed and my fear of open water pushed to the back of my mind, I was ready to travel to the Galápagos Islands to meet 200-year-old turtles that could teach us about ageing and sea iguanas that help save drowning children. It was March 2020 and with my passport in my bag and hope in my pocket, it was time to go. And then . . .

I should have been thousands of miles away in the Galápagos Islands, mirroring the footsteps of Darwin in the Ecuadorian sunshine. Instead, I was underground, in a bible-black Welsh cave, with a man called George. George did have a beard as strong as Darwin's, though, and was able to look into the distant past just like him.

The rude arrival of COVID-19 just a week before my trip stole day-to-day life from millions, including me. Over the next two years, the pandemic would bring darkness to my colleagues in the intensive care unit working at the coalface of medicine. Our faces would become coated in the dust of death.

With my travel plans cancelled and my diary filled with extra night shifts, I swapped my plane tickets for a crawl into an underground cave just a few miles from my child-hood home in South Wales. In reflected torchlight, my feet touched the ground exactly where another human had stood 20,000 years before. Our distant cousin had reached out their hand clutching a piece of flint and scraped on to the wall in front of me something important to them. Something they wanted to tell the world. Something that mattered. A picture of an animal.

And now 20,000 years later, in the midst of a viral pandemic brought about by the twisted relationship between humans and animals, I stood in that same place, staring at that same sketch – a beautiful reindeer with giant antlers, scraped into the rock deep inside the rugged Welsh coastline. It was some of the oldest cave art in the world, discovered by my archaeologist guide, Dr George Nash. He told me how the artist, likely a child using their right hand, had a deep understanding of the non-human animals they lived alongside.

Twelve hours later, I stood in one of the world's most advanced places in healthcare. And although I was no longer underground using a torch, I still used the deep understanding passed on from non-human animals to help save the lives of humans.

While the Galápagos Islands remained out of reach, I could visit Charles Darwin's English countryside home. Driving through the unusually warm British summer, I passed tiny villages with comedy names like Pratt's Bottom, before arriving at a grand, ivy-covered house. Darwin spent forty years living here with his wife and ten children, writing books that changed the world.

Inside the house, a small wooden cupboard under the staircase was filled not with boy wizards but tennis rackets. Above hung the only drawing from his 1859 book, *On the Origin of Species*: a branching tree, sketched in ink, tracing our distant family tree. Two simple words annotated the sketch – 'I think'. On the wall opposite was a map of the Galápagos Islands.

Walking through the manicured gardens, surrounded by beech, walnut and cherry trees, I found Darwin's 'thinking path'. This quarter of a mile track is where he would stroll and think and discover. It is where his books were written on the paper inside his head. It is also where Darwin developed angina before dying in his bedroom overlooking a mulberry tree. Listening to the birds, bees and aeroplanes as I walked, I saw horses and cows and a cricket match being played. It was an idyllic walk aside from the intrusive thoughts of Barry choking on a biscuit, the giraffe's neck and kangaroos' vaginas.

Although *On the Origin of Species* remains Darwin's most famous work thanks to it revolutionising our understanding of life, his second book, *The Descent of Man*, transformed the world once again in 1871. Darwin demonstrated that the difference between humans and animals is not one of kind, but only degree. In it he said: 'The love of all living creatures is the most notable attribute of man.'

Yet, our relationship with animals seems broken. The most time we spend with animals is when they are on our plate. We eat them and experiment on them. We keep them in conditions that destroys not only their wellbeing but human health and the environment. We blame them for pandemics and kill them for medicines that do not work.

But what if our relationship is merely cracked and not yet broken? What if individual humans are the problem and not humanity? And what if, by repairing our bonds, our shared lives can become better entwined, more beautiful and more noble?

This book hopes to fill these cracks with gold. To make the whole more beautiful. Each chapter will focus on creatures that live on The Land, The Air or The Sea. Then we will step below to The Underland, looking at death and everlasting life. Could listening to animals help us manage loss or even live for ever? Could it change the world for the better?

As another Welsh writer once said: 'We shall begin at the beginning.' Spinning the world on its axis, we will now first dive down under from the English countryside to Australia. Here we will see how the kangaroo's three vaginas can help us better understand the beginnings of human life. Join me on a journey to understand the lives and bodies of non-human animals. I want you to meet the patients I treat, tiptoeing along the shoreline between life and death. I want to share the science, the stories and the ethics of how we can save the lives of humans through understanding the lives of animals.

THE LAND

'A hundred lifetimes wouldn't suffice to see all the beauty in one acre of land.'

MARTY RUBIN

1

How to make a baby (kangaroo-style)

The cemetery was a strange place to think about vaginas, especially three of them. Surrounded by the concrete remains of life, we had come to visit the living rather than the dead. Almost-blue Australian sun scorched newly sprinkled grass. The minty zest of eucalyptus danced on the breeze. And there, in the distance, on top of a grave, two fat feet. Arms flexed like a middleweight boxer. Thick rounded hips like a wheel arch on an expensive car. And then – UP! Effortless bouncing, as if carried by an invisible stage wire. Bounce left, bounce right. A sudden stop at the lakeside, near delicate flowers laid on headstones remembering the once loved. Still loved. A mourner glances up with tears glistening on her sleeve; the sweat of loss.

We had travelled to Pinnaroo Valley Memorial Park in Perth, Australia, to see these bounding marsupials. It was not the kangaroos' jumping that kept my attention, but the tiny head of its joey just visible. Its head caught between the opening of the pouch like a nervous actor peeping through a stage curtain. And that joey had travelled through one of its mum's three vaginas. But why three? How? And could understanding kangaroo pregnancy help wannabe human parents like Lesley and John Brown once were? Let's find out by meeting their daughter, Louise Brown, the second person ever born without their parents first having sex. Although I'm unsure if Jesus really counts so she was likely the first. She was definitely the world's first test-tube baby.

Do you know the exact time and place you were made? Although birth stories are retold each time the smoke rises from extinguished birthday candles, conception often remains as it happened – under wraps. You may cringe at the thought of your dad ejaculating, yet what followed was the most important moment in your then non-existent life. You would become you.

Louise Brown didn't have to worry about such things. She sprung into existence on 10 November 1977 at exactly 11 a.m. in Oldham while her parents were 150 miles away in Bristol, witnessed by nurse Jean Purdy. No romantic dinner, no mood music, not even an orgasm. Although the media referred to Louise as the world's first 'test-tube baby', conception took place in a glass Petri dish. Two hundred and fifty-seven days later, on 25 July 1978, Louise Joy Brown was born at Oldham General Hospital by planned Caesarean section, weighing just 5 pounds, 12 ounces and an iconic image of Louise moments after birth, wrapped in a fluffy white towel, appeared on newspaper front pages across the world.

The first page of Louise Brown's autobiography, *My Life as the World's First Test-Tube Baby*, is profound because she dedicates the book to her four parents. Her mum, Lesley, was a very private person 'who ended up in the world's spotlight because she wanted a family so much'. After nine years of being unable to conceive naturally with her husband, John, due to blocked fallopian tubes, she underwent fertility treatment with Louise's other two parents, Professor Robert Edwards and Dr Patrick Steptoe. Although other women had been implanted with fertilised eggs before 1978, Louise was the first child to be born after this treatment. The Nobel Prize in Medicine was awarded in 2010 for this work.

Now that more than 8 million babies have been born using in vitro fertilisation (IVF) techniques since Louise, it is easy to underestimate what an iconic step in human history this represented. A Brown family photo showed the new arrival in a powder pink pram flanked by her parents in front of the iconic Clifton Suspension Bridge in Bristol. Three humans perched on the edge of the sheer Avon Gorge cliffs with the pinnacle of nineteenth-century engineering in the background. Bridges such as this one, which opened in 1864, demonstrated the Victorians' mastery over the natural world; in 1978 engineers of the human body had mastered life itself. They did so with the help of animals like the kangaroo that I was hand–feeding 15,000 kilometres away in Perth.

Kangaroos belong to the group of animals called marsupials, from the Greek word for the 'purse' in which these animals carry and nurse their young. Marsupials first evolved in South America 100 million years ago when the continent was connected with Australia and Antarctica. Today, Australia houses the largest number of marsupials with around 120 species, South and Central America having ninety species including the descriptively named elegant fat-tailed mouse opossum.

The first mammals were egg-laying creatures that didn't need to worry about embryo implantation. Eventually live birth evolved 160 million years ago in a common ancestor of humans and marsupials. Creatures like the kangaroo and opossum were the first to make the perilous journey from the deep, dark night of the uterus to the outside world as the first ever live-bearing mammals. Marsupial pregnancy, being at the crossroads of egg-laying and placental mammals, is key to understanding how the IVF techniques used to create Louise Brown were perfected. The adaptations needed to develop new life inside the body rather than in an eggshell were remarkable. We can now view the beauty of this process through tiny cameras inserted safely into developing embryos and by using detailed ultrasound scans that document life before birth.

The most incredible part of IVF, the creation of new life from a sperm and an egg, is the easiest bit. For some animals, fertilisation outside the body is just the way it is. Foreplay for the deep-sea anglerfish, the toothed seadevil, involves the male first biting the female, who is over ten times his size. After this romance is over, the male begins to fall apart, melting into his new mate until nothing exists of his body apart from his testes. The eggs are then released from the female and join sperm from the disembodied testicles. Fertilisation happens in the sea water all around. No hands to hold. The blue whale produces more than 400 gallons of sperm when it ejaculates. Perhaps one reason the sea is salty. With only 10 per cent making it into his mate, that leaves 360 gallons for the ocean. Another reason not to drink the salty sea water.

Knowing that external fertilisation was possible, scientists began to experiment with the creation of mammalian life. It is curious that the rabbit, known for its ferocious sexual appetite, was chosen as the mammal where fertilisation outside the body was first studied. Hungarian scientist Samuel Leopold Schenk showed that artificial external fertilisation in rabbits was possible in 1878, although artificially created human life would have to wait a little longer.

Imagine being the first person to actually see the creation of human life. Latvian-born Miriam Menkin was a highly educated lab technician working at the Free Hospital for Women in Boston, Massachusetts, in 1938. She was the first person to fertilise a human egg outside the body – a 'mother creator' of a new kind. Her weekly lab routine had remained constant for six years. Each Tuesday she carefully selected eggs the size of a full-stop from ovaries removed during routine operations. On Wednesdays, she would add a cloud of sperm to the eggs in a glass-bottomed dish. Thursday was a day of hopes and prayers before she peered down her microscope on Fridays to see if the egg and sperm had become a life. Six years, every week, the same outcome: nothing happened.

Yet one week, her familiar pattern fractured for the first time. After a change in theatre schedules, it was on a Thursday that Menkin selected an egg from a 38-year-old woman with four children whose uterus had prolapsed. It had been a tough week of sleepless nights for Menkin because her eight-month-old daughter had started teething. Through the sticky fog of tiredness, Menkin made an error. She normally mixed together sperm and egg for thirty minutes. Yet she was 'so exhausted and drowsy that, while watching under the microscope how the sperm were frolicking around the egg, I forgot to look at the clock until I suddenly realised that a whole hour had elapsed'.

Coming back into the lab on a quiet Boston Sunday morning on 6 February 1944, she glimpsed something that no one else had ever seen – early human life, shimmering through the bottom of a glass container. Two into one. It is beautiful that thanks to the challenges of caring for a young baby, millions of others can now become parents and live through these same struggles.

So why a gap of thirty-four years until the world's first IVF baby was born? The spark plug of life was never going to be enough without somewhere for the early embryo to shelter. Life needed to live back within the body but achieving this process of implantation and shelter was hard. Until we understood the kangaroo.

I've never enjoyed New Year's Eve. For a start the celebrations start way past my bedtime. Add to that the artificial construct of a new year 'starting' with a chime of a clock when time is just a continuous sea of change that laps at the edges of our lives. The drinks are too dear, the music too loud and the taxi ride home too elusive. However, had I been invited to the New Year's Eve party in London's Crystal Palace in 1853 my opinion may have changed.

Entering the vast Victorian skeletal building of Crystal Palace on New Year's Eve 1853, you would soon be struck by another skeleton. This one made of bone. Sitting inside were the most famous scientists of their generation, all dining within the bones of a giant iguanodon, the first full-sized recreated dinosaur. As they sipped on mock turtle soup, they sang these lyrics echoing around the bones:

The jolly old beast
Is not deceased
There's life in him again!
ROAR!

Sitting at the head of the table was Richard Owen, the man who gave dinosaurs, or Dinosauria (meaning 'terrible reptile'), their name. The creature in which they dined could easily have been mistaken for a giant kangaroo. That was because Owen, after first using frogs, then ostriches and other large birds as a reference, finally settled on the kangaroo as a model to base dinosaur recreations upon. The common acceptance that dinosaurs resembled and even acted like kangaroos stuck. Arthur Conan Doyle, known for his Sherlock Holmes stories, wrote *The Lost World*, published in 1912, in which dinosaurs jumped around on powerful hind legs, the forelegs folded in front of the chest. Dinosaurs were kangaroos with added teeth and scales.

Owen had a long fascination with what we now call comparative anatomy, examining the bodies of non-human animals to help him understand his own. He would often dissect animals that died in London Zoo, his wife once even arriving home to the carcass of a newly deceased rhinoceros in the front hallway. Following the voyage of the *Beagle*, Darwin had a large collection of specimens that Owen agreed to work on, including fossil bones collected in South America. Owen's later discoveries showed these extinct giant creatures were rodents and sloths, related to species in the same locality, rather than relatives of African animals as Darwin had originally thought. This was one of many ideas that later helped Darwin form his own concept of natural selection.

Owen's fascination with kangaroos started after seeing a tiny joey in the pouch, as I had in Australia. Finding out how it got there, he wrote in a Philosophical Transactions of the Royal Society of London paper in 1834, was 'an inquiry well deserving attention'. Leafing through the yellowed pages of the original manuscript shows us for the first time pencil-shaded drawings of life's machinery inside this hopping creature.

Through Owen's work, we know the kangaroo's three vaginas are used for different purposes – two for having sex and one for giving birth. This arrangement is shared by other marsupials including koalas, wombats and Tasmanian devils. The two side vaginas carry sperm to one of two uteruses while the middle vagina is how baby joeys exit to the outside world. This strange set-up is matched by a two-pronged penis in male marsupials.

Like most quirks of nature, it bears evolutionary advantages. While adult kangaroos can be taller and heavier than the heavyweight boxer Muhammad Ali, joeys are born just the size of a jellybean to help fit into the cramped innards. Joeys are extremely immature when born. From a selfish gene's perspective, this allows the female kangaroo to remain in a cycle of perpetual pregnancy. One tiny joey in the pouch plus an embryo developing in the uterus, while an older child can continue to be nurtured in the outside world – three for the time price of one. Life can sometimes be a game of numbers even if it's not played with dice.

However, it is not the visible organisation of the kangaroo's reproductive system that has informed successful human IVF, but rather the features that cannot be seen. After the mystery of external human fertilisation had been solved with the help of rabbits, the next challenge was to implant the new life back inside. This is where marsupials helped to lead the way.

Kangaroos and rabbits were not the only animals to help humans become parents. For decades, the most accurate pregnancy test sounded like something out of Harry Potter. British biologist Lancelot Thomas Hogben imported thousands of African clawed frogs in the 1930s after working in South Africa. The 'Hogben test', at its peak carried out tens of thousands of times in Edinburgh, involved injecting urine into the skin on the back of the frog. If the frog laid eggs by the next day, the owner of the urine was pregnant. It wasn't until the 1960s that the modern pregnancy tests used today, based on antibody technology and not frogs, were introduced. Seeing that line appear on a pregnancy test is always a special moment, now replaced with the clarity of a digital word saying PREGNANT – although being told by a frog that your life is about to change has more poetry to it. Eight months after Lesley and John Brown saw their own special line, the world was about to change as an artificially created human life took her first breath.

The big leap forward was the ability to safely implant their embryo inside Lesley and convince her body to accept the alien invader. If the Moon landings were the greatest exploration out of this world, a baby born through artificial insemination would easily match this achievement inside our world, inside the human body.

Although poetic in many ways, we now know the first part of the embryo to develop in the womb is the end, or arsehole. Basically you were once just an arsehole. Some people never change. Then, soon after, you develop extra lizard-like muscles in your hands. These are one of the oldest memories of our evolutionary past, seen in humans dating back to more than 250 million years ago when we changed from reptiles to mammals. Although lizard hands have few uses today, these early changes made our thumbs dextrous by keeping an extra muscle, unlike our other unopposable fingers. But before getting to this stage, life needs to burrow into the lining of the womb, to implant, to stay safe for nine months. How?

In humans, 75 per cent of unsuccessful pregnancies are the result of failures of implantation rather than fertilisation. Only after this essential step can the embryo start to develop. Making life is easier than keeping life. Loss of a child, even one that is still a foetus, is an ageless plight. Millennia of loss has not dulled this emotion. For parents dealing with early pregnancy loss, it is a particularly cruel type of death, one that is hard to quantify. It was the potential rather than the actual that carried so much joy. What would they be like? Who would they be? You will never know.

Our loss came when our future child turned eleven weeks old. Just days before, the screen of the hyper-white plastic ultrasound scanner had been filled with grey pixels of life. A tiny heart, the size of a pea, squeezing out blood the size of two human tears on every beat. A tinny speaker in the machine shouted out a swooshing noise for every heartbeat, the same sound you hear when your own heart beats against your eardrum at night.

Days later, a small bleed, a return trip to that same scanning machine. Now the pixels stayed still. Silence said so much. A tiny heart the size of a pea. No longer squeezing out blood the size of two tears every beat. One for my wife, one for me. The future felt grey, the world coloured like cement. Hope become a memory. It felt like we would never again walk on the sunny side of the street. But we would.

This early stage of pregnancy has a lot in common with a twisted knee. Emergency departments often meet people in their forties who develop knee pain after playing an unexpected game of football. In their mind they were still that fit, athletic teenager, yet their body was more realistic and creaked with every kick. A sudden twist, a swollen knee, painful and red – the cardinal signs of inflammation. Inflammation is also key to a successful pregnancy – at the start during implantation and in childbirth at the end.

It was long known that following implantation, the lining of the uterus would switch to an anti-inflammatory state to prevent rejection of the foetus. After all, the embryo is a mismatch of genetic material, as foreign to the body as an infection. Too much inflammation in early pregnancy can result in miscarriage, just like when the body tries to expel an infection. Therefore, researchers had experimented with drugs and procedures to dampen down the immune system in cases of recurrent miscarriages or failed implantation. Little were they to know that putting up a little fight was helpful to sustain future life. Clenching your fingers improves grip as well as makes a fist.

It was through studying pregnancy in marsupials like kangaroos and opossums that helped us understand why suppressing inflammation by taking drugs like ibuprofen can actually lower rather than improve human IVF success rates.

Conversely, scratching the human uterus to cause inflammation may increase implantation success, giving life to children like Louise Brown.

Before studying marsupials, doctors saw implantation as a one-sided process, the responsibility only of the early embryo attaching and embedding itself into the uterine wall. It seemed IVF could only be successful with improved embryo quality. We now know that like all relationships, it needs to work in both directions. Implantation is a complex process dependent on both the foetus and the mother.

We discovered that embryos in animals like opossums are initially still covered by an eggshell. Yet for the placenta to form, this shell needs to break. The mother's body gently eats this shell, producing digestive enzymes that dissolve the calcium carbonate material, the same substance used to make blackboard chalk. This digestion prompts an inflammatory reaction that damages the lining of the uterus. This inflammatory stage can also contribute, along with hormonal changes, to morning sickness. This slight damage promotes implantation and placental development, which were the steps that most challenged early IVF and led to early pregnancy loss like we experienced. Just as the swollen knee needs that swelling to heal, life too needs adversity to thrive.

IVF doctors can now use several molecular markers derived from understanding these clues left by marsupial pregnancy to help detect receptivity to implantation. This can allow the timing of embryo transfer to be just right to allow implantation. The use of inflammation as a form of communication between mother and baby is truly special, with echoes from our marsupial past. We now know when drugs like aspirin and ibuprofen can be safely used to help foster rather than threaten the nurturing home for an embryo.

All parents know that pregnancy is only the start of the journey for both them and baby. The birth of Louise Brown was remarkably straightforward. The Caesarean was swift and smooth, the baby healthy and that baby is now a mum to two children herself. Yet for millions of babies around the world, the transition from inner womb to breathing air is too much. They need help from the outside world as soon as they leave the inside world. Next, we will meet my good friend Lucy, her husband Owen, and their children. All three of them. The triplets. Although born much larger than the jellybean-sized joey, they needed more than a pouch to survive. They would need luck, medicine, but also touch. At just the right pressure. Like a monkey. But first, let us go to the jungle.

2

ROCK-A-BYE BABIES

The petrol-fed motorboat arrived like a wasp landing on a red flower. The crooked smile of yellowed teeth from the driver welcomed us like sunshine on an autumn day. Life jackets handed out like sweets from a packet. My young daughter slipped in her arms, drowned by the oversized floats stuffed into the outside pockets. The speedboat bobbed, the water lapped, the anticipation was building. We travelled through the humid, sweat-soaking air on the speedboat-bobbing sea around the floating village of Kota Kinabalu and then on to Sepilok to meet our long-lost family. Long lost. Still lost.

Welcome to Borneo, where orangutans swing and groom each other and teach us how to live better. We were hoping to see the old man of the jungle in Borneo's twisted tree roots, a family of orangutans with a new orphaned baby girl called Chikita (meaning tiny). Chikita was one of the smallest babies that has ever been rescued by the Sepilok Orangutan Rehabilitation Centre and introduced to a new adopted family to care for her. These orange ancestors of ape can teach us how tiny human babies can be kept alive despite being born months too early. Chikita would show me how the power of touch is powerful indeed. Neonatal intensive care units have just learnt the lessons these animals have long known. And Chikita's adopted mum would remind me how a new human mum once cared for her own babies with similar grace despite millennia of separation from her primate past.

A newly-wed couple, a farming business, a decision to start trying for a baby. To start. The first month, she was late, the test was taken. Two solid lines mark the strip. Pregnant.

My friends Lucy and Owen went to their first pregnancy scan soon after my wife and I had lost our baby. The ultrasound started, cold gel on to soft skin. Searching for the new life began: a heartbeat, beating strong, a child. But soon Lucy heard that same long pause of silence that we had. Her silence, though, was different, not tinged with sadness or with loss, but with gain. Not one heartbeat, but two. Then, not two heartbeats. Three.

'I need to get my boss,' said the sonographer. 'Nothing's wrong, I just want to check something . . .'

The drive home through the Welsh twisted lanes back to the family farm seemed to take much longer than ever before. Lucy practised aloud what she would say to family waiting on the doorstep.

'The scan was fine. Everything's okay.'

And it was in many ways. Many ways. It was fine, but it

was fine not for their one baby, or their second baby, but for their three babies. Triplets. Natural triplets. The first month of trying. They started trying and stopped all in one.

Pregnancy was hard. Reflux, no sleep, worry about what was to come. Twin girls inside next to one boy. Two eggs had been released that month. One split into two to make identical twin girls. One remained intact to make a boy. But 2 + 1 still = 3. And all three needed to come out and survive. Around a half of twins and nearly all triplets are born prematurely before thirty-seven weeks. Although the kangaroo's jellybean-sized joey is born after just thirty-four days, for most of history humans did not have a pouch to care for premature babies. Lucy worried about how her children would make it safely from the protection of her body to the outside world. She worried about their ability to care for more children than their hands could even carry. She worried how they could get through this unscathed.

Premature birth still kills many babies and affects one in ten pregnancies. Despite advances in the care of premature babies, those born before twenty-eight weeks and weighing less than a pineapple have only a one in two chance of survival. They often need help breathing, eating, fighting infection and staying warm. They need help to simply live and grow.

The neonatal intensive care unit has technology to help support these vulnerable lives. Better breathing machines were developed in the 1970s, then new drugs to improve the elasticity of their tiny lungs in the 1990s, and then a decade later came steroids drugs to further help. However, only in the last ten years have we learnt about the power of something that every parent can do to help their children – the power of touching them.

Used alongside conventional neonatal treatments, so-called 'kangaroo care' encourages parents to hold and touch even the most critically ill premature babies on life support machines. Parents' skin touching baby's skin. Skin to skin. This improves their chances of survival by a third. Babies that are held suffer fewer infections, have better temperature control and less lung disease. Being carried and touched helps them gain more weight and even grow in length and head circumference. Although called 'kangaroo care', this medical innovation has more in common with the parenting styles of our distant ape ancestors. It should perhaps be renamed 'monkey care'. The ways that primates use touch socially will help explain how Lucy's hands could help her babies survive. It may even hint at why humans laugh at jokes, party and take drugs. The mother and baby orangutan I was about to meet in Borneo, despite not telling me any jokes, had been practising these techniques for millions of years.

We walked through the forest floor, the debris of life forming a dense carpet of vegetation. My cotton shirt was saturated and I felt beads of sweat slide down my back like a kid on a waterslide gaining speed before splashing on to the waistband of my shorts. Our local guide strode ahead effortlessly; long, slender brown legs, like driftwood. His face scored with lines, one for each time he had walked through this jungle he called home. Then a crack. A snap. Branches sway without wind. They bend down as if praying, then flick back to shape as an amber blur moves across. Orangutan Mum emerges from the blur of branches, her back carrying the precious cargo: Chikita, her daughter, just weeks old.

Orangutan is one of those beautiful words that describes perfectly what it means. My native language, Welsh, does this too. Grandmother in Welsh is mamgu, translated to 'dear mother'. Anaesthetist, ceidwad y cysg, 'protector of the sleeping'. Peach, eirin gwlanog, 'woolly plum'. Orangutan, 'old man of the jungle', in Malay.

Chikita's fingers wrap around coarse hair, her legs knotted to Mum's body like a wrestler, toes crunched together gripping as hard as her hands. You too may grip just like Chikita. Open your human palms now, pointing upwards towards the ceiling. Make a fist and then bend it inwards towards your body. Look at the lines of tendons from the base of the heel of your hand travelling towards the middle of your forearm. Some of you will have two lines, two tendons. But some of you will have three, an extra tendon attached to an ancient ape muscle called palmaris longus that was helping Chikita grip tightly to her mum's back.

I stood there for almost an hour by myself. Not lonely. Just alone. Mum and baby Chikita lay down on the ground, Mum's hands searching through her child's fur for bugs that were not there. As she did, another adult orangutan stood behind her, mimicking the same actions, grooming the mother, touching her back, stroking her hair one way and then another. Forming a line, they searched each other's fur for bugs that were not there. They touched, they groomed, they bonded. Thousands of miles away, Lucy held the smallest of her triplets born at thirty weeks, the little boy, Joe, in her arms. Joe's cheek pressing against her bare chest. She stroked the papery skin on his back with her index finger of one hand. With the other hand, she ran a fingertip slowly from shoulder to his wrist that was still speckled with blood from medical tests. She rocked back and forth, singing the lullaby her own mum had once sung to her.

Lucy didn't know it, but she was following an ingrained behaviour from our primate past. She was grooming Joe like Chikita's mum. She touched, groomed, bonded. But why? Why do apes and young mothers groom? Why should it help tiny babies survive?

To bring these apes of the past together with tiny human babies today, we need to think about gossip, small talk and grooming. After first meeting a monkey on his East African garden veranda aged just three, British anthropologist Robin Dunbar came to study the behaviour of primates through his love of human relationships. He grew up in a scramble of cultures where African tribes, Arabic and Indian communities lived as one. Speaking Swahili as a child, he wrote poetry in Sanskrit and only got his first real job aged forty. Living in the world of Empire gave him a never-ending interest in human interactions.

Despite his early meeting with monkeys on the veranda, Dunbar had little interest in wildlife. Friends and family saw animals only as targets down the end of a rifle. Dunbar came to animals through his love of human behaviour, unlike other primatologists such as Jane Goodall, who learnt about human behaviour through her first love: animals. After being turned down for a post as a clinical psychologist in London for out-publishing his boss, a chance encounter with baboons on a university expedition to Ethiopia sparked his interest in primate behaviour. Studying their watchmaker fingers delicately folding coarse grey hairs from one side to another like a hairdresser perfecting a parting, Dunbar questioned why primates spend so much time grooming. It takes them away from finding food, leaves them open to predators and takes a lot of energy. Dunbar wondered if grooming may influence how big a primate community could grow and spent the rest of his life trying to find out.

This wasn't time wasted. Dunbar was right. The set group sizes that baboons live in are replicated throughout human society from the Russian army to Italian mountain villages to Welsh rugby teams. This magic number could even help medical teams better work together. But for now, how can primate grooming, like that between Chikita and her mum, save the lives of premature babies like Lucy's triplets?

The touch of another human can reduce stress in adults as well as babies. In an experiment by a university in North Carolina, participants watched a romantic video with their partner, followed by some having a twenty-second hug. They were then given just two minutes to prepare and record a speech, which was played back to them. Designed to be a stressful experience, the blood pressure and heart rates went up much less in participants who had hugged.

Around the corner from where this experiment was done, a human hug resolved a potentially deadly situation during the 2020 Black Lives Matter protests.

'Tactical vehicles, armed officers in riot gear, the crowd uneasy. Of course, there's yelling and screaming,' said one officer during a standoff between armed police and a crowd of increasingly agitated protesters in North Carolina. Then, in an astonishing moment, sixty of the armed police officers kneeled in solidarity with protesters. Moments later, the lead protester, with a bright red bandana, moved forward and hugged the officer in charge. The next day, a newspaper front page featured the embrace with the protester's tears rolling down her cheeks on to the officer's bulletproof vest. The standoff was over. The tears shed were the sweat of love sealed with a hug.

Touch can even give us mind-reading abilities. A simple hand placed on the arm can convey a range of emotions that can be read by total strangers. In another experiment, after having their arms stroked, pressed or squeezed, participants could correctly identify the expressed emotion 80 per cent of the time, from anger to fear, disgust to love, gratitude and even sympathy.

It shouldn't be a surprise that touch is important to human development. The grainy pictures of impoverished Romanian orphanages, where the only contact was with metal cot bars, document lifelong developmental problems when human touch was out of reach. Throughout the COVID-19 pandemic, our loss of touch was like living in a time when the crusts were cut off the sandwich of life. So, too, if you stop apes grooming, they quickly become low, sad and ill. So just as touch can bring health, robbing us of contact or feeling touch can lead to problems, as Johnny Cash will now show us.

Life comes around like a big vinyl record. The days are long, the years short. One minute you are a son or a daughter, the next a mum or a dad. I can still smell the damp air from my childhood garage where my dad would play me his favourite records. After the Beatles, the Who and Dylan, we would finish with Johnny Cash before my mum called us for dinner. Through the scratches of the monophonic vinyl player, the trumpets announcing the start of his song 'Ring of Fire' would always make me smile. Thirty years on, I now play my two girls Johnny Cash songs in my air-conditioned car in high-definition surround sound. They still sound as good.

It is hard to get old without a cause, but Johnny Cash

had his wife and his music. At the age of seventy-one, with serious health problems, Johnny Cash's voice trembles as he opens his powerful cover of the song 'Hurt', released in 2002. The accompanying video, recorded in his home of thirty years, flicks between the glamour of his surroundings and Cash's fading health. His square hands creak on a guitar, disfigured and old. Although the lyrics were written seven years earlier by the youthful American rock band Nine Inch Nails, they speak to Cash's struggles. It talks of needles tearing holes, of pain and of sadness.

Cash was suffering from the effects of long-term diabetes that had destroyed the nerve endings in his feet, his hands and even his spinal cord. He needed to inject insulin into his thigh three times a day. The high levels of sugar in his blood had frayed the very nerve endings that respond to the light touch used in both primate grooming and premature baby stroking. Losing the feeling in his feet meant even a grain of rice in his shoe could cause a severe injury. Not feeling that subtle rubbing of the skin while walking could lead to a minor skin sore. Not feeling the minor skin sore would lead to a bigger sore and then an infection. The nerves affected in Cash's spinal cord meant he suffered from the painful condition of autonomic neuropathy. His nervous system would go into meltdown at the smallest insult, making his blood pressure skyrocket, his skin sweat and his heart rate become erratic. The song 'Hurt' was so powerful because it was sung by someone hurting.

Despite Cash's musical resurgence, his ability to perform was stolen by the pain from his diabetes. Then his wife,

June Carter Cash, died. It is hard to get old without a cause. Closing the piano with his painful hands in the final scene of the video was a prelude to Cash's death just seven months later. His last words were rumoured to be 'I hear the train a comin'.'

After years of research, Dunbar has shown that rather than removing bugs, the main purpose of grooming in primates is to make and keep social connections. These develop not just through psychological bonds strengthened by spending time together, but through hardwired connections between touch and the brain. In the womb a foetus is thought to experience touch before it can hear, smell or taste. As the pregnancy progresses, twins even reach out to touch each other. What can apes tell us about this touch?

Special receptors in the skin of monkeys fire only when activated by light touch at the exact speed found in grooming. Too hard and they do not respond. Too fast or too slow and they do not respond. But light touch at exactly three metres per second sends impulses from the skin to the spinal cord into a primeval part of the brain. There, brain cells release chemical messages, including endorphins like serotonin, dopamine and painkillers as strong as heroin. There is a direct link between grooming, touch and the brain chemicals that cause happiness and pleasure and love. Alchemy for the soul through the hands of others. Chikita's mother was hot-wiring her child's emotional system by using her fingers while also maintaining social connections with her wider group.

We now know that these same nerve fibres are found in humans and tiny babies like Lucy's triplets. Her motherly instinct to hold and to caress and to stroke facilitated releasing powerful chemicals in the brains of her babies. Studies in neonatal intensive care units have shown that babies who are touched and stroked need fewer painkillers to safely stay connected to life support machines. Lucy was providing nature's heroin, happiness and love to her children through her own hands. Through her own touch.

But how can this also explain Lucy's rocking and her lullaby? Dunbar realised that as families and communities grew in number, there would not be enough hands to groom everyone. Yet keeping social connections remained essential. Loneliness is a cancer that may kill as many as smoking and obesity. How can loneliness be avoided when touch is not possible or not enough? Are there further lessons from the larger community that Chikita belonged to that could help human communities all over this big blue marble we call Earth?

Grooming takes time to be done well and there are only so many hours in one day. Therefore, evolution produced either small group sizes or else promoted abilities that were more scalable than one-on-one grooming. Speaking with Robin Dunbar, his eyes widened before he laid out his theory of how larger groups maintain their connections. 'The answer must be language. Grooming with our mouths replaced touch with our hands. Words instead of fingers.'

The evolution of language in humans, Dunbar argues, allowed group size to increase, yet the benefits of grooming to be continued. Small talk, gossip, even feasting, rituals and comedy would slowly replace the role once played by our hands. In time, other brain-altering chemicals, such as psychedelic drugs and alcohol, would complement our voices to replicate the effects of touch on our brain chemistry.

Amazingly, the same nerve fibres found in the skin of primates and humans are also found inside our ears. These sensors respond to low-pitch noises, in slow cycles the same speed as mothers rock their babies. Lucy's movement, sensed by her babies' inner ears, fires off those same receptors as her touch. A nursery rhyme's pace, the rocking, the stroking – all throwbacks to our ape ancestors grooming for bugs. When you have too many backs to scratch and not enough hands to do so, you instead use music and dance.

Perhaps this is why we nod our heads to good music, why humming vibrating mantras is such a powerful tradition. It explains why humans have large bulging pieces of overgrown bone behind our ears called the mastoid, perfect for reverberating low-pitch noises, despite their tendency to get infected and cause illness. Perhaps this was why, on my wedding day, I cried not at the speeches, nor at the sight of my beautiful wife, but when I heard the Welsh male voice choir sing 'What Would I Do Without My Music' in their low-pitched, vibrating, slow rhythms.

3

WHY YOU SHOULD EAT SHIT

I can't remember the most important day of my life. Neither can you. It has been said that the two most critical days are the day you were born and the day you realised why. Although we have all been born, of course, not all of us know why just yet. Although you didn't get a slice of cake on your birth day, many of you will have eaten a mouthful of something much better for you – shit. Happy birthday to you.

The most likely position that you exited from a vagina was occiput anterior or, put crudely, your mouth facing your mum's bottom. With contractions as strong as a small elephant standing on your foot, it is entirely normal during labour for faeces in the rectum (lying just behind the womb) to be squeezed out. The result is a mouth full of poo as a 'hello world'.

Although unpleasant to read, this gift is actually a gift of life. Your first meal was teeming with biological life, containing more species of fungi than stars in the night sky. It is also a gift of health – babies born facing their mother's bottom have lower rates of diabetes, asthma and eczema than those born facing the front or by Caesarean. To understand why, we will return to Australia before heading to the world's largest beer festival in Germany. But first, let's catch up with the triplets born months too early and now struggling to survive.

The triplets were not given the gift of faeces on their zeroth birthday as they were born by Caesarean. Seconds after being flashed in front of Mum and Dad, they were whisked away to the sterile sugar-white surroundings of the neonatal intensive care unit. Born at just thirty weeks, their tissue-thin lungs were too young to breathe without help, their skin too fine to keep them warm. Instead, they relied on a human-made kangaroo pouch of plastic – an incubator and a life support machine.

Their immune systems struggled to deal with the millions of bacteria that live on the hands of even the cleanest nurse. Joe, the smallest of the three, struggled the most. Weighing the same as a pocket dictionary but with far fewer words of hope held inside, his oxygen levels were dangerously low late one night. A plastic tube, the thickness of dried spaghetti, had to be punctured through his translucent skin, draining air that had leaked between his lung and ribcage. Days later, the skin around this tube glowed red. Weeping and sore, it had become infected. Joe looked like a broken bird lying on his back, every need attended to by machines.

The infection spread through Joe's blood, causing his

body to shake. Lucy and Owen would also shake each time their phone rang. They feared any news from the hospital would be the worst kind; they worried they would have to swallow the darkness. But, thanks to powerful antibiotics, Joe pulled through. He did have hope written on the inside after all. But no sooner had his skin infection receded, a new problem emerged – from his bottom in bouts of bloody diarrhoea.

Tests showed that Joe had a bug, different to his skin infection, that caused the lining of his bowel to become inflamed and sore. The bug was called Clostridium difficile, also known as C. diff, an infection caused by the powerful antibiotics that had just saved his life. To understand how modern medicine can now treat C. diff, we must first dive inside our inner ecosystem of bugs that we all nurture. We will find life growing inside our own stomach, meet the world's oldest caterpillar and eventually eat shit.

As my computer screen flickered to life, I saw beautiful aboriginal art hanging on the wall behind the Nobel Prize winner and doctor, Professor Barry Marshall. Our video call was streamed from his remote 200-acre farm in the Western Australian outback. He was destined to become a doctor specialising in the gut – his mum a nurse and his dad a chicken factory engineer on the outskirts of a gold-mining town. Infections in the factory commonly caused outbreaks of bloody diarrhoea in chickens and then humans.

Marshall told me he once treated an elderly Russian man, suffering from a terminal stomach condition, with antibiotics in desperation. Weeks later, the Russian returned to the clinic completely healed. 'He was practically doing somersaults into the consulting room!' said Marshall. 'The antibiotics shouldn't have done anything, but they did.'

In the 1990s, Marshall's outpatient clinics bustled with patients and their ulcers. Even water samples from the River Thames in faraway London had high levels of antacid drugs, so common was their use. Despite these treatments, many ulcers would slowly erode through the lining of patients' stomachs. The only treatment left had been removal of the diseased parts of the gut.

When checking for cancer in these surgical specimens, Marshall and his pathology colleague Robin Warren kept seeing the same strange twisted black shapes deep in the stomach lining. It was odd to see life surviving in such acidic conditions. Thinking back to his Russian patient cured by antibiotics, Marshall wondered if stomach ulcers could be triggered by an infection. Were these spiral black lifeforms the cause rather than the result of disease?

Marshall read old reports of cats, cows and dogs having similar strange findings in their gastric lining. These findings had been ignored by human doctors and their significance unknown. When he told colleagues about his ideas, they laughed him out of the room. The idea was just too weird. And it was weird. Marshall was questioning the accepted view that bad diets and stress caused ulcers. Marshall couldn't be sure he was right, but the doubt persisted. It was a ghost in the fog. But uncertainty is strangely the very best way to motivate progress in medicine and science. Every answer starts with a question. Every question starts with someone admitting I don't know. So Marshall dusted off his instincts and set to turn I don't know into now we know.

Marshall hatched a cunning plan. After putting a camera down into the stomach of yet another patient with an ulcer, he kept a cup of juice (vomit) from the inflamed stomach. Marshall grew the bugs present in this fluid in his lab, noted what antibiotics killed them, before putting his theory into practice. Leaders must often make whatever horrors exist concrete. Only then can they be broken apart. Swirling around the patient's vomit, he tipped the cloudy broth into his mouth, closed his eyes and swallowed.

'My stomach gurgled, and after five days I started waking up in the morning not feeling good, and I'd run to the bathroom and vomit,' he told me with a slightly crazed chuckle.

Marshall repeated the camera test this time on himself and saw, in all its inflamed, red and angry glory, a damaged stomach lining, just like his ulcer patients had. If it had been caused by bugs in that vomit, the antibiotics Marshall then took would help. Should help. May help. May not. If not, perhaps he too would need an operation.

Weeks later, his self-inflicted ulcer was gone.

Today, his colleagues still laugh at him. Not because he was wrong, but because he was right. So right that in 2005 the Karolinska Institute in Stockholm awarded the Nobel Prize in Medicine to Barry Marshall and Robin Warren for their 'discovery of the bacterium Helicobacter pylori and its role in gastritis and peptic ulcer disease'. It was the same type of bacteria that had been found in cats, dogs and cows decades earlier.

Recounting the story, Marshall said: 'Obviously, if you think too far out of the box, you're very fringe – and I say the only difference between a genius, eccentric and someone who's mad is that someone who's eccentric has money.'

At the end of our call, I asked Marshall about the aboriginal art hanging on the wall behind him.

'Oh that's not art, that's my own stomach lining infected with the Helicobacter pylori bug that caused my ulcer!'

The discovery of H. pylori in humans led to a revolution in the treatment of ulcer disease. Now, as well as new antacid medications, antibiotics form a key component of treatment. Removing parts of the stomach, a common operation just twenty years ago, is now rarely done. If tuberculosis was a poster child disease of the nineteenth century, H. pylori was the model in the twentieth century.

Being so ubiquitous, H. pylori may be the most successful bacterium in the world. The bug was found in the mummified remains of a South American woman clutching her two small children from AD 1000. Five thousand years ago, a man was shot by an arrow and clubbed to death in the European Alps. Called the 'Iceman' after being mummified by a glacier, H. pylori was in his stomach contents too. Using genetic diversity data, researchers have created simulations that indicate the bacteria had spread from East Africa around 58,000 years ago. Marshall even thinks H. pylori may have caused Charles Darwin's recurrent bouts of vomiting on board the *Beagle* long before it set sail to the Galápagos.

Its success may lie in the secret advantages that the bug gave its users. People colonised with H. pylori are almost half as likely to have asthma or allergies. The bug produces folic acid, an essential vitamin for people who would have been living on limited diets during the agricultural revolution of the past.

These advantages must have extended not just to humans. Decades before the Nobel Prize, it was known that other animal species had stomach linings infected with this bacteria. Almost all domesticated cats have H. pylori infections, likely the cause of so-called 'fur balls'. Lions have harboured the identical strain of H. pylori as humans for tens of thousands of years, which begs the question: Did we get the bug from lions or them from us? Who ate who?

The failure to link animal and human disease slowed the development of an effective treatment for ulcer disease by decades. The discovery of H. pylori also started a revolution in our understanding of how external life, living inside us, can affect our health. But before you think about drinking someone's vomit, let us instead travel to Germany and drink beer. Then we will meet the world's oldest caterpillar, who strangely has no bugs living inside it at all.

Thick sounds from brass bands vibrate inside my bone marrow. German sun flashes against the shining blond metal of instruments. Oversized chiselled glasses filled with amber beer clash and clink and spill. No one cares. Liquid splashes, people stand, arms stretched above in worship to the song. Music is the operating system of the human soul tonight. Beer is the fuel, borrowing happiness from tomorrow. The tent's ceiling is painted powder blue with fluffy white clouds yet stars hang from tense wires. Sunshine and night-time together. Through the fabric door of the tent, a buxom woman swings a long mallet through the air, crashing down on an old fairground strength meter. Bell clangs, a prize, a wide smile.

I had travelled to the 'village of 6 million people', the capital of Germany's Bavarian state, Munich. Although Oktoberfest, the world's oldest beer festival, first held in a fairground in 1811, was one obvious reason for this trip, I had actually come to see something very different. And much older. Forty-four million years older.

The next day, beer still on my breath, I tried to make friends with the morning. I set out to meet the world's oldest caterpillar, preserved in Baltic amber the same colour as that beer, in the Bavarian State Collection of Zoology. Embedded in amber, sleeping, untouched, safe. The length of a grain of rice, it had been crawling on the bark of a tree 44 million years ago, the same time as marsupials were evolving in Australia. Trapped by the glue of tree sap, it became frozen in time, perfectly preserved, until human scientists found this time capsule.

I had travelled to Munich not to wonder only at the age of this caterpillar but rather to wonder at what it lacks. Unlike most other animals, the guts of caterpillars, including 44-million-year-old ones, contain no other bacteria other than what they have just eaten. This needs an explanation.

Professor Barry Marshall, through drinking his patient's vomit, showed how the life continuously bubbling inside humans can have a dramatic effect on their health. Although some bugs like H. pylori can cause disease, millions of others do not. Instead, they are essential for health. We call these inner microbiological passengers our microbiome – the genetic mass of bacteria, fungi, protozoa and viruses that live inside or on our body.

Despite adverts selling harsh chemicals that 'kill 99 per cent of germs dead!', our nearest neighbours will always be microbes. Our skin is covered in them, our mouths are their home and our clothes partially made from them. They are our smallest enemies yet our most important allies. The bugs on your skin help break down ammonia into sweat, release chemicals that help lower your blood pressure. The bugs in your mouth produce nitrates that prevent oral cancer. Farmers have lower rates of rheumatoid arthritis due to the constant swirl of bugs on their hands, in their food and in their lives, keeping their immune system busy and out of trouble. We don't even know yet what the 140,000 viruses living in our gut do.

More than half of your body is not human, with 57 per cent of your cells actually being microbes. And they are arranged in ways just as complex as the astronomical constellations. Your faeces are not one amalgam of dung, but have a complex layer structure. If you were to uncurl a poo on to a plate and cut it in half, it would be like the world's most complex layered dessert cake from a fancy French patisserie. The outer layers closest to your bowel wall harbour bugs that tolerate oxygen. As we dive deeper away from the surface, the bugs become more anaerobic, finding oxygen toxic. Your poo is a dynamic, complex life form within your own life form, changing with time and environment and health. Yet only now are scientists starting to ask: what would happen if we changed our own microbiome?

Although our guts are home to 90 per cent of our microbiome, life lives everywhere the air can touch. We have friends living on our eyes, ears, nose, mouth, vagina, anus, urinary tract, armpits, groin, between our toes and in our belly button. The number of genes from these bugs is 200 times greater than those in our own human genome. If removed, your microbiome would weigh the same as twenty blueberry muffins. The exact combination of these bugs is as unique to each person as a fingerprint.

The microbiome seems ubiquitous. Humans and most other species rely on billions of these tiny organisms to digest material, extract minerals and even produce vitamins. Some have even crazier uses. The bobtail squid harbours one species of glowing bacteria in the area between its eyes. They produce an eerie green glow, like a head torch, thought to help the squid search for food. The light produced also acts as an internal timepiece, dictating sleep and wake cycles like an alarm clock embedded into its head.

However, the caterpillar's inner life is different. Compared with other animals, caterpillars have 50,000 times fewer microbes.

'If human guts are like a rainforest in terms of microbial abundance, caterpillar guts are like a desert,' says the world expert on caterpillar poo, a rather niche position.

Why would this be? We have seen how important the microbiome is for health so why would caterpillars dispense with their best friends living inside?

For caterpillars, there must be a high cost to having a resident microbiome. Bacteria compete with their host for nutrients and can aggravate the immune system just like in ulcer disease. Caterpillars manage their herbivorous lifestyle by eating massive amounts of plant material and may have little need for help. Plus, their short, simple gut structure is a bad place for millions of different bugs to call their own home. Its simplicity means fewer niches and crevices for bugs to specialise into.

Applying lessons from this 44-million-year-old caterpillar to humans, we see our microbiome has a cost when modern medicine gets involved. The antibiotics given to tiny Joe to treat his infection worked but had other consequences. As well as killing the bugs making his skin glow red, they destroyed the delicate balance of his gut's microbiome. Some bacteria, including Clostridium difficile, became dominant, causing a second life-threatening infection in Joe's bowel lining.

How could we redress this balance of bugs? The caterpillar refreshes its mix of microbes every time it eats but it couldn't be that simple for Joe, could it? Are there other animals that reset their microbiome when things go wrong? Can they hint at new treatments for humans like Joe? We need one further animal to help us solve this puzzle. Let's return to Western Australia and find out why their very cute koalas need to eat shit.

Just a thirty-minute drive from Barry Marshall's Australian farm is the family parkland reserve of Yanchep. First used as hunting grounds by the First Nation Noongar people, now all that is hunted are ice creams by visiting children and flat whites by their tired parents. My family had travelled along a sand-dusted, pastry-coloured road to glimpse Australia's favourite cuddly toy, the koala. Although widespread across the continent, Western Australia lacked koalas until 1938 when a colony was introduced to Yanchep. After a tough few years of chlamydia infection outbreaks, the colony of eight were now visited regularly by tourists on a boardwalk around the park. We were those tourists.

The splintered timber underfoot creaked as we neared a toffee-stuck huddle of people all pointing in the same direction. We had driven in sweat-soaked clothes with our young teething daughter to see something we hoped she would love. And finally, there, at the end of the pointing people's fingers, was the bundle of fur with a stoned, cartoonish face we had come to see.

'Look, Evie!' I exclaimed. 'Koalas!'

'. . .'

Nothing.

The koala is the link between the sterile gut of caterpillars and our overpopulated bowels. A 5kg adult koala eats over half a kilogram of one of the 800 species of eucalyptus every day. The types of toxins in this high-fibre, low-protein plant varies by region across Australia. And it's thanks to the koala's microbiome, with bacteria species that neutralise these regional toxins, that they can survive.

As we circled the boardwalk, our toddling daughter's reaction started literally as a bored walk. Then came the screams with a bright red face meaning one thing – time to bribe her with food. At the time she was weaning from milk to solids. We would spend hours blending organic fruits and vegetables for her to spit on to the floor. A few years later, those first-child best intentions would be replaced by Happy Meals and potato waffles. The weaning experience for the koala we were watching had been just as organic but very different.

A young koala drinks its mother's milk for six months while living in her pouch, developing eyes, ears and fur. At six months weaning begins but with no organically blended fruit in sight. Instead, nuzzling around the mother's back end stimulates production of liquefied faeces, appropriately called 'pap'. This gruel-like slurry contains unique bacteria that breaks down toxins found only in the local eucalyptus species. Koalas give their offspring a faecal transplant, a ready-made microbiome, perfectly balanced to help their young survive.

When koalas were first imported to Yanchep, their microbiome mix was not designed for the local eucalyptus species. The keepers, remembering how koalas are weaned, hatched an ingenious plan to allow the new arrivals to adapt to the Western Australian eucalyptus. They collected faeces from koalas living near similar species in other parts of Australia. They packaged this poo in acid-resistant capsules and fed it to the new imported koalas. Sure enough, the microbiomes of the koalas changed, allowing them to safely digest the local eucalyptus. The zookeepers' knowledge of eating shit allowed them to pioneer faecal transplants that decades later would be used in humans.

At the start of this chapter, I described your first-ever meal as a gift of life from your mother shortly after birth. It has now been shown through clinical trials how the mixture of microbes inside your gut can have a radical impact on health. Although this is a modern concept in medicine, it is old news for koalas, who have known for the past 40 million years.

The Caesarean that kept Lucy's triplets safe had also put them at risk. Without the gift of life from Lucy's own microbiome, the smallest baby, Joe, was left struggling with a severe bowel infection. One microbe called C. diff became dominant, causing life-threatening bloody diarrhoea. Until a few years ago there was only one treatment – more antibiotics.

But the caterpillar and then the koala have shown us how to balance the bacteria in our gut. The caterpillar shows how the microbiome can change and adapt according to environmental inputs. It purely takes on the microbial pattern of the food it eats. The koala has shown how even in more complex animals this is possible and such a change can lead to real health benefits. We now know the microbiome is a dynamic and changeable inner life form. Nobel Prize winner Barry Marshall showed we can change the bugs inside us to help treat disease. And so too did the Australian koalas near his farm, importing a new microbiome.

Joe's doctors were increasingly worried that his infection was getting worse. Although they didn't know it, they needed help from our animal past. Could they change Joe's microbiome? Was this even possible? One final trip, this time to Boston, will tell us.

If you ever find yourself short of money on the pleasant, walkable streets of Somerville, Massachusetts, you have options. This suburb of Boston is forward-thinking in a number of ways. In July 2020 it became the first US city to legally recognise polyamorous relationships. Partly to allow the visiting of sick patients during the COVID-19 pandemic, homes with more than one 'loving partner' now have rights similar to married couples. Somerville also boasts a large red-brick building, appropriately opposite an all-you-can-eat buffet restaurant, that stores 25,000 frozen shits.

After eating Boston's famous baked beans, just hand over the resulting product directly from your bottom to the not-for profit company OpenBiome. You give them a plastic container containing your poo and they give you $60. Your faeces will then be mashed in a blender before any undigested food (sweetcorn, no doubt) is removed using a metal sieve. The mush is spun down in a centrifuge and the anti-freeze glycerol added. A quick plunge in liquid nitrogen results in a frozen faecal suspension that is just as effective as fresh faeces for treating C. diff and can be stored for two years.

Stool banks are the result of research showing infections like C. diff can be treated using human faecal transplants. Studies from a stool bank in Birmingham in the UK show transplants are more effective than antibiotics, with an 80 per cent cure rate after just two shots of frozen faeces are squirted through a plastic tube in the nose down to the stomach.

It was hot July sunshine that first welcomed the triplets home. Driving down the rubble path to their farmhouse, the yellow rapeseed waved like a carpet of Brazilian flags. After a month in hospital, Elsie, Grace and their little brother Joe were home, carried in all bundled up in blankets by Lucy and Owen. The antibiotics had finally treated Joe's C. diff infection just as the doctors were awaiting arrival of frozen donor faeces.

Years later, Joe had become the largest of the siblings.

Harry Potter obsessed, he once treated his sisters to a surprise extra-short haircut without his parents knowing. He would tear around Ikea with my own children, shooting a bow and arrow down aisles over the heads of passers-by.

Lucy had originally worried about their ability to care for more children than their hands could even carry. She had worried how they could get through unscathed. Yet they did. Adrenaline, love and hope was their fuel. And double espressos. The early days were hard, the later days even harder. They cried but also laughed. Did they come through unscathed? No. But most of the scars were ones that healed and reminded them of what they had achieved. Life was never the same again. Some parts worse, most parts much better. And better thanks to understanding the inner world of their microbiome, life inside life, lessons passed down from koalas to tiny human babies.

4

HEAD IN THE STARS

Today started at 5 a.m., the neon blue of the morning light barely breaking through the velvet black of the wide African sky. Breakfast was black coffee like no other. Rich, bitter, sweet. The beans that were crushed to wake me up did not come by air or by container ship. Instead they travelled by truck over the red dust and crusted salty roads of Kenya's Central Highlands. The water that washed the toil from the workers' hands came from the Riara River, fed by highland mountain streams.

I had travelled to Empusel (literally 'the salty, dusty place'), in the heart of Kenya, known more commonly as Amboseli National Park. A dry cradle of Africa's human history, still filled with game animals, Maasai tribes and safari vehicles. I was here on honeymoon, my mind filled with love and not with death. Yet a decade later, meeting Ifan in an intensive care unit would send my memory straight back to this dusty place. For it was in Kenya where I gained the knowledge that could help to save him.

It didn't involve understanding a machine, a drug, or even a human.

Our white safari van bounces along, holding on to the corners of the track like a drunk sailor gripping his boat. Dust hangs on to hot haze. Trees fly past the scratched window, flattened green tops, held by twisted wood. The sky seems too big, stretching out across the arc of the African flatlands from right to left, from front to back. Brakes are pressed, arms brace hard, dirt rises.

'Shhhh, look! There!'

And there, standing. Matchstick legs rise into powerful, curved hips. A long, slender tail, with patterns that fade into soft black brushed ends. Densely patterned skin, a kaleidoscope of yellow sandy roads covered in chocolate-brown butterflies. That muscular body hides a 25-pound heart, pumping 60 litres of blood every minute. Pressing, squeezing, twisting. The unseen red blood rises, skywards, as the pressure builds so it can reach the brain, 2 metres above. The Maasai giraffe turns, and looks down. I look up in awe.

Seven million years ago, on the woodlands of Eurasia, lived the giraffe's last common ancestor, Samotherium major. This bull-like creature used its metre-long neck to eat both tree leaves and grass. The continued elongation of the neck by natural selection, resulting in the 2-metre neck we see in modern giraffes, was accompanied by further anatomical and physiological adaptations.

The number of bones in the necks of birds, reptiles and amphibians varies considerably. Gaze over Lake Nakuru in the Rift Valley of Kenya and your eyes see a landscape filled with the marshmallow pink of 2 million flamingos, each with nineteen neck bones. The ducks whose brown feathers fleck the pink carpet each have sixteen, while geese have between seventeen and twenty-three neck vertebrae and swans more than twenty-four. All mammals, apart from sloths and manatees, have just seven regardless of the length of the neck, including the giraffe. Although the simple concept of longer neck equals more leaves to eat, this extreme adaptation places huge burdens on three systems – the brain, the lungs and the connective tissues.

The variations in nature's machinery are interesting to explore. However, consider them against the backdrop of human disease and they offer novel approaches to how we treat medical problems. Much in today's understanding of how human brains respond to injury, and even how we save the lives of people with asthma, can be traced back to how a giraffe's body works. The giraffe can even show us how 'intelligent design' is not so clever.

We approach the cracked mud walls of the village. A young boy, maybe three years old, carries a scruffy goat in his arms. A strange mangle of noise travels through the thick scorching air.

Beautiful, powerful, uneasy.

A background drone plays like a bagpipe, with melodic voices calling out, answered in return by a crowd. Smoke rises from a fire somewhere. I feel like I am in a huge football stadium, surrounded by chants and music and sweat and drums. Here lie hundreds of years of music theory smashed into one. The Maasai welcome song welcomes me to their village and into their lives.

The Maasai chief is at the front of the group; bright red robes wound around skinny body. Hundreds of tiny beads, strung into lines of colour, hanging from ears and mouth; years of life scratched into the deep creases in his leathered skin like grooves on a record. Then the jumping starts.

The village warriors form a tight circle. A young man moves into the centre, legs delicate like the giraffe's, narrow and straight. With a bend at the knee, he flies up higher than should be possible, again and again. Only his toes touch the flaked-scalp ground before another launch. As he reaches the top of his ascent, the singing pitches up, louder and higher:

> *'I the warrior of the long thin spear*
> *Am not at all arrogant*
> *But a humble being whose neck is weighed down*
> *   by poverty*
> *Poverty of a herd that falls below fifty.'*

Six thousand miles away, a decade after my Kenyan honeymoon, I meet Ifan, a nineteen-year-old student. The Western society in which he had grown up was radically more modern and advanced than that dusty Maasai place. Yet tribal violence remained. Walking home with friends on a chilly January night, Ifan would find those darkest hours that come just before the dawn.

Five young men walk towards Ifan. Anger, conflict and

red run through their veins and through their brains. Short words are exchanged. Fists tighten. Fight? Or flight?

'I don't want to fight,' are the last words Ifan will speak for weeks. The men attack, a heavy blow to Ifan's head with a traffic cone. Feet kick and hands punch. Blood runs. Ifan's hard skull hits the harder edge of a concrete kerb. A broken skull, a bleeding brain, a build-up of pressure inside. Police later find drops of Ifan's blood on the road, on the window of a house and smeared on a parked car – the bloody signature of violence stretching some 50 metres. Six months later, a courtroom is shown a pair of trainers, poorly hidden under a bed, stained with Ifan's blood. Justice is finally done.

I met Ifan lying deeply unconscious in a hospital bed, having hundreds of years of medical theories and treatments thrown at him. Doctors hoping he will live, nurses caring, family praying. They use the knowledge they have to help his brain – to give it enough blood by increasing his blood pressure. Do not let the pressure inside his skull get too high. Allow used-up blood to leave. Keep the level of gases in his body just right. This knowledge has been handed down through generations of scientists and doctors. Yet the giraffe I saw through that scratched safari truck window has known what to do for 7 million years. Although its brain is healthy, it still needs enough blood and a pressure that is exactly right. Can it teach us how to better care for Ifan?

Although a giraffe's long neck is its most striking feature, what happens inside its body is even more remarkable. Its brain, perched those 2 metres high above its heart, needs the same amount of blood per gram as a human brain just 45cm above the heart. Place your fingers on the side of your neck, pressing against your firm corrugated windpipe. You will feel the regular tapping of your carotid artery knocking at your fingertips. This is your blood, squeezed out from your heart. The dense muscle contracts, twists and pushes it to every part of your body.

If I were to pull out a Maasai hunting sword from its cattle hide scabbard and swing it through your neck, your head would start to tumble towards the floor. Before it gets there, a column of blood would rise nearly a metre above your severed neck. This flow is enough in health, but after Ifan's brain injury, the pressure from extra blood and swelling inside his skull was building. Scottish scientists in the nineteenth century taught us that the bony skull is like a rigid box. Pressure building up inside prevents enough blood from moving in. To counteract this, we can remove parts of the skull using drills or else push blood in ever harder like the giraffe. The 100mmHg of pressure in Ifan's healthy arteries was no longer enough to push blood to every injured brain cell. A giraffe's blood pressure is also insufficient to reach its brain. So how do they manage?

The Maasai giraffe walks slowly from low scrubland to lush green. Foot first, then leg, the body follows like a catwalk model. Birds dart by in a rush of feathers. I start to imagine what is inside this creature's body.

Thud, thud, thud.

The huge heart muscle pounds in my mind. Thick red muscle, double the width of Ifan's heart. A human heart this size would soon fail, and the person would die. Oxygen would be unable to get through the thick layers from the outside to the inside. A heart attack would then follow. Yet giraffe hearts stay healthy. They have lower rates of heart disease compared with most other mammals. Why? How? We don't know. We haven't even asked until now.

The heart needs to be fillet-steak thick to push the deep red blood up so high. Up, then up, then up even more. A giraffe's blood pressure is double that of a human: 200mmHg. Giraffes have the highest blood pressure of any animal. This pressure is enough to push blood to the tip of its brain, just like Ifan also needs. When heart specialists examine their hearts, giraffe's ventricles are extremely thick without the scarring or fibrosis that occurs in people as they get older. We now know this is thanks to mutations in five genes related to fibrosis, which may have important benefits in human disease. Their hearts are also wired differently, allowing more time for these chambers to be filled, helping eject even more blood.

After eating from the tree, the giraffe moves again. Water, like silver foil, is just visible in the distance. Legs stride, with purpose yet no rush. The 6-metre-high tongue moves towards the ground. A slow angle of the neck down towards the land, like a tall fishing rod, arrow straight, eased towards the surface of the sea. As the animal lowers, gravity pushes vast amounts of blood from body high, downwards towards the earth. As the brain dips below the body horizontal, the pressure inside the skull should become extreme, as with Ifan. Yet the giraffe's body knows that too much venous blood pooling is bad. Instead, the giraffe's blood vessels are lined with strong one-way valves preventing blood from rushing downhill to its brain. The water is cool like autumn rain.

When I meet a critically ill patient following a brain injury, I now know what treatments may help thanks to studying these adaptations from the giraffe. As Ifan lay unconscious, plastic tubes were inserted into veins in his neck. These would carry powerful drugs to make his heart squeeze harder and faster. Instead of a double vodka volume of blood squeezed out every beat, his heart would now push out the equivalent of three shots.

His blood pressure would be raised from 100mmHg to as much as 180mmHg using these medications – nearly as high as a giraffe's. Pressing in blood harder would counteract forces inside his head opposing this flow. As well as making sure enough blood gets in, we also ensure blood can leave. The bulging neck veins seen as singers reach a high note can be squashed by clothing or medical equipment. Lacking the valves a giraffe has, blocking these soft floppy tubes would prevent blood returning from the brain to the heart, increasing the pressure inside even more. We loosen Ifan's clothing, we push his blood pressure higher, his brain responds and comes slowly back to life. But the danger is not over, for Ifan or the giraffe.

That cool drink on the savannah does not last long. A bush moves, the dust rises. A dash starts, animal chasing animal. The long, lumbering giraffe moves at surprising speed. The adaptations needed to do this lie skin deep. These same techniques now allow a fighter pilot to break the sound barrier without passing out. How?

In what feels like another lifetime, while training as a doctor I joined the Royal Air Force. I thought I was destined to become a military medical officer, to fight and to defend. Aged just nineteen, signing wet ink on to thick parchment in an oak-lined military base, the excitement of promised adventure eclipsed the loss of autonomy that I would feel five years later.

This sense of entrapment came as I drove a shiny blue sports car, bought with the spoils of my cadetship, towards a military base to start officer training. My life was now committed to another cause. I could not turn around, even if I had wanted to. And I did want to.

I had changed as a person since that 19-year-old signed his name. I had just got married. My wife, a teacher, wondered where I would be, where she would be and how life would change. And the only honest answer I got from senior officers, understandably, was 'we don't know yet'. To some, that uncertainty is exciting. And it was to me, yet the inability to choose the eventual outcome was also terrifying. As I drove, I lingered on the fact that I could not turn around. Not if I wanted to remain in the military.

And then, I turned around.

I pulled on to the side of the road, called the base and said: 'So sorry. I won't be there today, or ever. Sorry.'

I left the military before I had really begun. For some, quitting is a cowardly move. For me it was the bravest thing I had ever done.

Although I never saw active service, my time in the military had some real highlights. The highest, literally, was learning to fly. Sadly, my last ever sortie before parting left a bad taste in my mouth – vomit. Having learnt the basics of taking-off and landing, one sunny morning my Navy fighter pilot instructor 'Ratty' (not his real name, I hope) decided to put the textbook lessons aside. He wanted to show me his signature acrobatic move known as the 'Ratty Roll'. This consisted of a series of sharp angular turns that contorted my insides like someone had inserted a food mixer through my belly button. The final twisting of the aeroplane applied just enough gravitational force to drive any remaining blood from my brain, deep down to the soles of my sweating feet. I experienced tunnel vision, or gun-barrel vision, as my brain was starved of blood.

Then through fanned fingers I vomited all over the cock-pit, which only made the distribution of sick even more unfortunate.

Landing minutes later, almost translucent, I was handed a bucket of water and a toothbrush. Not for my teeth, but to clean every tiny button and switch in the aircraft.

As the giraffe gallops across dusty ground, the hyena pack quickens. Tongues out, backs arched. Yet they struggle to gain as the 5-metre giant hits 60km/h. The sheer forces on the giraffe's long limbs are immense, but so too are the adaptations needed to keep blood flowing sky-high to a brain moving significantly faster than Usain Bolt. If blood went to the giraffe's feet as gravity had intended, the heart would be empty, nothing to squeeze to the lungs to pick up oxygen and no oxygen to go to the brain. The animal would, like that younger version of me, develop tunnel vision, feel sick, vomit and then faint. It may die. The hyenas would have lunch, and dinner, and breakfast the next day. Yet they do not eat. The giraffe runs, outpaces, escapes, lives on. How?

In 2017, Nasa awarded its highest recognition, the Distinguished Public Service Medal, to Alan Hargens, a professor of orthopaedic surgery. The forging of this medal started during a trip to Africa in 1985 where he noticed that young giraffes could walk as early as one hour after birth. Further research showed this was due to blood vessels in young giraffes' legs quickly thickening. Not only did this help stability but prevented their high blood pressure causing profuse bleeding from minor leg injuries. Deep under the skin of their legs, giraffes have tightly wrapped fibres, squeezing down on blood vessels like a compression bandage stopping them bleeding. The same idea would later help astronauts survive space travel.

These adaptations to deep skin layers in giraffes also explain why they do not faint when running at such high speeds. Many animals have skin of different thicknesses in their various body parts. The reason CEOs can walk on hot coals during overpriced team-building days is not mindful-ness but the 2cm thick skin covering their heels. If the coals were placed on their tissue-paper-thin 0.05mm eyelids, there would be fewer high fives in the bar afterwards.

Giraffes have remarkably thick skin around their legs and neck, combined with thick, elastic collagen fibres. This skin is dense and tight, like a wetsuit that clings to every ripple of your body after a winter of eating. As blood rushes towards the feet during a hyena's chase, the giraffe's skin fights back, squeezing blood up to the heart in time with each gallop. The faster the run, the harder the squeeze in a beautifully efficient feedback cycle.

Alan Hargens and his colleagues at Nasa realised the potential of this super-stretchy skin for 'gravity suits', clothing to help fighter pilots and astronauts maintain their circulation while battling extreme gravity. If I were allowed back into the air with Ratty, this time in his Navy F-35, we could be travelling at 2,000km/h, 1.6 times the speed of sound. My body would be contorted by seven times the gravitational force on Earth, equivalent to Apollo 16 re-entering our atmosphere after landing on the Moon. Without the lessons learnt from our Maasai giraffe, I wouldn't just be sick, I would be dead. The lack of blood supply to my brain would soon render me unconsciousness as I entered 'G-Lock'.

To prevent this, pilots now wear powerful pneumatic trousers that squeeze the blood vessels in their legs, stopping blood from flying down into their feet, keeping their brains fed with oxygen and keeping them alive. Even without hyenas at their ankles, fighter pilots and astronauts can fly high over the plains of Africa thanks to space medicine technology found on those dusty ageless savannahs below.

The hyenas hang back, pacing around a broken tree like troublemakers around a park bench. They stare at the horizon, glance down at the empty ground. The giraffe, safe at distance. But only just. The hyenas had been outrun. But only just. The giraffe had slowed down, not because its legs were tired or its energy depleted, but because of a whirlwind of air. This twister was not circling through the outside dust but inside the giraffe's own windpipe.

And so, too, was Ifan dealing with problems in his own breathing system. Lying still in an intensive care bed, Ifan's lungs were now causing as much concern as his brain injury. Now doctors struggled to push enough breath into his body to keep the levels of carbon dioxide stable.

To understand how we helped Ifan, we need to explore how a giraffe can breathe through such a long, thin neck. And to understand this we must travel back to the 1940s and sit in a British Cruiser tank on the battlefield of the Second World War. There we will meet a marvellous man – Dr Philip Hugh-Jones. He would become a leading chest physician and one of the most important clinical scientists in post-war Britain. He was also obsessed with animals.

'My dad loved to take medical students on a ward round to London Zoo,' his son, the anthropologist Stephen Hugh-Jones, told me over a cup of English breakfast tea, sitting in his Welsh cottage home.

'The students got quite a lot out of it,' I later read in an interview with his father, 'I mean the bright ones. The stupid ones just thought it was a day at the zoo. There are few people who have a chance of looking at an elephant's or tiger's eye fundus.'

Stephen's dad had initially wanted to do zoology. Instead, after studying medicine at Cambridge during the Second World War, he was sent to investigate the effects of tank fumes on soldiers' bodies. This sparked his early interest in chest medicine and a move to my hometown of Cardiff, Wales. Some worried that the 'black gold' of coal flowing out from the gritty Welsh valleys was affecting the lungs of miners. Dr Hugh-Jones would eventually prove this to be true, describing the disease pneumoconiosis or 'coal-miner's lung'.

Downtime between his ground-breaking research studies was spent in a home filled with art and with music, with pythons and rare butterfly-breeding experiments, surrounded by strange antiquities from faraway places. Rather than a cat or a goldfish, their pets included a sloth called Sophie and a bush-baby named Tuppence, who enjoyed nothing more than peeing over the bathroom floor.

After my tea, Stephen offers some wine. He recalls his childhood in Jamaica where his dad first classified diabetes into types 1 and 2. Yet, alongside these world-leading breakthroughs, his son's education was more grounded.

'My school in Jamaica taught me about sex, swearing and throwing stones across vast rivers,' he describes with a nostalgic smile.

Yet these lessons contributed to Stephen's great achievements in javelin on return to an English boarding school, as well as his lifelong passion for anthropology.

'As an anthropologist, I now study sex and swearing as a professional rather than as an amateur!'

It was during another overseas research trip that Dr Hugh-Jones made a breakthrough we could now use to manage Ifan's wheezy lungs. Spending time with the remote Maku tribe in the Upper Amazon, Dr Hugh-Jones saw prey caught using poison-tipped darts, sent flying by a swift breath into a blowpipe made from hollowed out stems of a palm tree that grows dead straight. The taller the tribesman, the longer their pipe. The longer the pipe, the further flew the deadly dart. Yet there was a limit to the length of bamboo that sent darts any further – too long and the dart barely fell out from the end, like the final drops from the wine bottle in Stephen's house. Tribal elders explained that when the 'breath' inside the pipe exceeds the breath in the mouth, the pipe is too long. The taller the blower, the more 'breath' they have.

What this age-old tribe was describing neatly fits the research findings that Dr Hugh-Jones would describe later in his career – lung volume is directly related to height. However, it would take a chance meeting with a giraffe years later to show Dr Hugh-Jones why the length of a blowpipe is so limited by these factors.

On one occasion during his famous London Zoo ward rounds, a giraffe sadly died after emergency surgery on an injured foot. As part of the post-mortem, Dr Hugh-Jones was pictured measuring the 1.7-metre-long giraffe's windpipe. Thinking back to the blowpipe limits, he wondered how giraffes could ever survive with such a long breathing pipe. Could the explanation from tribal elders also apply to living creatures? After additional measurements were made, he found the answer. Through millions of years of natural selection, the giraffe's trachea had become much narrower than any similar species, reducing the volume or 'dead space' inside. Unlike the Amazonian blowpipes, this allowed a giraffe's windpipe to exceed the length imposed by physics.

After completing his measurements, Dr Hugh-Jones found a 4-metre-long string-like structure. One end attached to the giraffe's brain, then threaded down the long neck for 2 metres, around a large blood vessel, only to return 2 metres back up to the voice box. This tissue, shown by Richard Dawkins on Channel 4's *Inside Nature's Giants* in 2009, was the recurrent laryngeal nerve, which co-ordinates the movement of the vocal cords in mammals. Through a random quirk of early embryological development, this nerve takes a route to the voice box around a small arch of tissue during foetal development. That small arch soon swells into the largest blood vessel in the body, the aortic arch. In humans, by adulthood the nerve's detour path is hardly noticeable, adding just a centimetre to its journey. Yet in the giraffe, the nerve is pulled upwards the entire length of the neck, 2 metres in one direction, only to dive back down 2 metres in the opposite direction due to the tangle. You would have to be very generous to describe this as intelligent design. It would be like me wrapping an electric extension cable around my entire house twice just to cut the grass on my front lawn.

But Dr Hugh-Jones's work was not finished. By attaching soft tubes to the nostrils of giraffes and camels, carefully closing one side with his hands at a time, he described how breath flows through these narrow tubes.

Giraffes take very deep yet slow breaths to combat the dead space in their tremendously long, narrow trachea. The flow in these pipes during calm breathing is smooth, like a tap running half open. Yet due to the narrow diameter, when breathing becomes faster, the flow becomes rough and turbulent, like filling the bath with taps fully open. Our giraffe had to stop running at top speed from the hyenas as this turbulent airflow had started.

Forty years after Dr Hugh-Jones held that giraffe's trachea to the sky, Ifan's asthma now benefited from this knowledge. Back in the intensive care unit, we first removed any connecting plastic pieces between Ifan's lungs and the life support machine. These are detachable pieces of dead space, not contributing to gas exchange and reducing the efficiency of each breath. Like the giraffe, we increased the volume of each breath and reduced the number of times Ifan was breathing every minute. He would now breathe like a giraffe, slow and deep, allowing him to keep running from his own predators, his assault days ago still afflicting his brain.

5

THE AN(T)SWERS BENEATH YOUR FEET

I hate flying, but love travelling. It's a sacrifice I happily accepted to exchange the headache-grey British October sky for the incense-tinged sunset of Bali. I'd been asked to speak about this book at the biggest festival of words and ideas in South-East Asia, the Ubud Writers and Readers Festival. The theme that year was karma. It took about six seconds to compose the thirteen characters needed to reply to the invite: 'I will be there!' Some decisions are easy. Yet on the sixteen-hour flight I faced a much harder decision, one that would shape the rest of my life.

'Do you want the chicken or vegetarian meal, sir?' asked the flight attendant.

There was an awkward pause. It felt like I had waited a lifetime to answer this question. I kind of had.

Flying across the equator flips your life. Through the aircraft window I peered down at how the moonlight reflected on the land. The same lunar glow as seen from my homeland, but different. A half-Moon, now drawn from left to right like a wide smile, not from top to bottom like my Moon. Rows of oil rigs dotted the Persian Gulf, churches of the sea worshipping black oily magic.

Time. Passed. Slowly. Everything on the aeroplane was a clock – the film that dragged, the crying child, the bags under my eyes that grew.

'Sorry sir, chicken or vegetarian?'

My mind jumped helplessly to an essay I had written twenty years ago while at medical school: 'The vegetarian vivisectionist – can vegetarians experiment on animals?' I dug out the yellowed pages of my thesis when I returned home, the final paragraph read: 'I truly believe that vegetarianism is a moral requirement of the majority of the human population. This can be logically argued alongside the justification for the use of animals, where no alternative exists, in cases where it will be certain to safeguard human life. Having come to these conclusions, I must either embrace a vegetarian lifestyle or else embrace moral hypocrisy. I fear that, with gustatory reluctance, vegetarianism shall have to be my path.'

For twenty years I had remained a moral hypocrite. The flight attendant was still there. Unhappy.

'Chicken?' she suggested firmly.

It seemed strange to fly halfway around the world to speak about the wonder of animals after eating their flesh. And for what? A nice taste?

'Vegetarian please.'

Only twenty years too late.

And then it was morning. Bright, almost transparent. I

squinted through the window over the wing. We descended towards the rolling swash of sea. Headphones away, passport in hand, teeth brushed but my mouth remained stale. But not because of any chicken between my teeth this time.

Soon I unfolded on to my hotel bed. I felt like a broken bird. But tomorrow would be worse. Tomorrow I would be viciously attacked by an animal. Hardly karma. But this tiny animal will teach us how to care for a broken Ifan, who remained in hospital, critically ill.

We left young Ifan after his street assault, fighting for life with a severe brain injury. His fight was made easier by a giraffe that showed us how to better care for asthmatic patients like Ifan by using long, slow, deep breaths through our life support machines. Days later, another disease knocked on the door. This time Ifan developed a severe infection.

Caring for critically ill patients often requires plastic pipes to be threaded through blood vessels into cavities deep inside the body. Sometimes my job feels like plumbing, although any leaks are of the thick red liquid of life. Sadly, blood is also a great place for other life forms to grow.

Even though Ifan was normally a fit teenager, becoming critically ill left his immune system vulnerable to invaders. Bugs may have got in through his delicate lungs, or the plastic tubes we inserted, or even through the wound left on his head after brain surgery. But once the microbes drank nutrients from his blood, they multiplied again and again and again. They replicated exponentially, each generation a doubling of the last. Within eight hours, even a single bacterium could produce 1.5 million new cousins. After one week with infinite resources, there would be more bacteria cells than stars in the universe.

And so it was no wonder that Ifan's body struggled to fight this rampant infection. His temperature shot up, burning like cheap tobacco, his heart raced, his organs started to shut down. Despite receiving the strongest antibiotics, his infection continued to worsen. His brain was now not our main concern, it was the rest of his body. After racing to hospital by moonlight one difficult night, we told his mum and dad that Ifan was sick enough to die. We didn't know what else to do. But a tiny ant did.

Waking through the haze of jet lag on my first day in Bali, I tried to force the new time zone into my body. The heat stuck my cotton shirt flat against my back as I drank a thimble-sized glass of orange juice before going to get another from the breakfast buffet at the hotel.

Ubud is the cultural heart of Bali, a kind, vibrant, alive, flower-filled town of 100,000 people. Walking down the brown dusted cobbled streets outside my hotel, mopeds blurred past like wasps. Their engines sang against the background hum of birds and chickens and humans in a chaotic chorus of real life.

My ageing bones ached after the long flight; my back arched down towards the ground. So the neon sign directing me towards a traditional Balinese massage parlour felt like karma. Soon I was wearing just my boxer shorts beneath a napkin-sized towel, lying face down on a shaky raised bed. Glimpsing through one eye, I saw my thick-set masseur, smiling yet ready for business, rubbing together strong oiled hands.

'What pressure would you like, Mr Matt? Soft or firm?'

There could only be one answer. 'Firm,' I said, firmly.

Perhaps it was my Welsh accent, but he must have thought I had actually said: 'Like a fat elephant standing on my back in stilettos please.' Because the next twenty minutes of my life was spent trying not to scream or cry.

It wasn't the first time I had been professionally massaged by a man. Years ago in India, I had a traditional Ayurvedic massage by a guy with a gigantic moustache. It mainly involved pouring oil down my arse crack and was a strange experience, one that I would rather not repeat.

Although I felt comfortable with my current masseur's biological sex, I had read in the flight magazine that, shockingly, being gay in Bali at that time was illegal and punishable by imprisonment. So too was pornography or even being provocative in public. That was when my irrational mind started playing tricks.

As overwhelming pain shuddered through my bones on each firm stroke, I became increasingly anxious about turning over. The more I tried to concentrate on not getting an erection, the more I feared what would happen if I did. I rehearsed the phone call to my wife from the prison in Bali: 'I didn't mean it, but I turned over and had a semi. Then the police arrived.'

Thank goodness, after twenty minutes lying face down, the ringing of a delicate bell signalled the treatment had finished – without a jail sentence. Getting up from the bed, I had bitten my lip so hard to endure the pain, there was blood on the towel underneath my face, which I quickly stuffed in my bag while getting changed. It is fair to say I felt much worse than before I went in.

'How was it, Mr Matt?'

'Oh, just wonderful, thanks!'

Apart from the pain, towel theft and constantly thinking about being imprisoned.

That evening, I tried another method to ease my body. Walking through the terraced rice fields around Ubud, I stumbled upon a yoga studio. First opened on the Day of Happiness in 2004, it was run by Sheila Burch, a Californian who had first come to Ubud in 1985 while travelling the world. The pull of the people, the place and the peace meant she stayed permanently.

As I walked up the rich wooden staircase of the open-plan building, the view from the yoga terrace was stunning. Endless tiers of rice fields folded out like layers on a green wedding cake. Joining me that evening were a handful of backpackers, exuding youth in their sweat. Our instructor looked like the resident cat (called Kucing), toned, a wide smile and even wider legs as she laid on the floor in full splits.

'Namaste, welcome,' she said with a knowing, hushed tone.

The backpackers put their hands together like they knew what they were doing. I fumbled with my water bottle, spilling it on the floor.

'First we will do some introductions,' said the instructor.

'I want you to tell me your name and how you are feeling this evening.'

'I will start. My name is Nina. This evening I am feeling "changeable" because I am having my period.'

'I am Noah,' said the handsome one with long hair. 'I feel grounded.'

'Tabatha. I am feeling humbled,' said the one who had been eating pomegranates when I arrived.

I went last. 'I'm Matt. I feel old and stiff.'

What happened next is hard to recount. It was like a cat contortion competition where I was an old salty sea dog. In some positions, I thought I had it right and felt great. Then I would look across at the oversized mirror where, staring back at me, was a sweaty Mr Bean playing Twister. The degree of my limb movements was barely measurable and my Downward Dog looked more like a Drunken Donkey. And then the hiccuping began.

But just as I felt like an impostor in my own body, I looked up at the sunset that had quietly arrived. The sun was dripping over the horizon, the grass in front of the yoga studio now illuminated by a thousand fireflies. Suddenly, I fell a little bit in love with Ubud. A year later, the chemical illuminating those fireflies would be used to test for a disease no one had yet heard of – COVID-19.

Along with the fireflies, another creature arrived right on cue. The wooden floor under my feet was covered by a puddle of sweat like there had been a raincloud over my head only. Walking with purpose towards this salty lake was a perfect single file line of giant wood ants. As the final pose was made by Nina, her foot high on her opposite leg like a stork, one of the ants crawled up my leg. Probably attracted by the massage oil from earlier, it dived under my shorts. As the group all placed their hands together and said 'Namaste', I was frantically fumbling with my hands down my pants.

Despite this momentary inconvenience, ants just like these could help us treat Ifan's severe infection. They are still helping us find new antibiotics, teaching us how to better use the ones we already have and can even show us how to protect others from pandemics like COVID-19.

Forget nuclear war, meteor strikes or pandemics, antimicrobial resistance is the most pressing global threat of our time. And it has already arrived in my hospital, in yours and in everyone's. These indestructible bugs live on the doors to the clinically clean operating theatres, the toilet seats where the surgeons sit to check their email and even on the skin of the nurses who clean the scalpels.

The speed that infections can resist antibiotics now

outstrips the development time of new synthetic drugs. This isn't just theoretical. Although Ifan was given the best antibiotics we had, his infection was getting worse, and we had no alternative treatments. Yet there were answers closer than we thought, just under our noses, if we had kept our noses closer to the ground.

In the time it takes you to read this sentence, 700 million ants will be born. Ants had been on our planet for 100 million years before we arrived. They have civilisations as complex as early humans', with division of labour, hierarchy and even public health systems. African Matabele ants carry injured colleagues after battle back to the nest to tend to their wounds. They have a triage system: dying ants aren't treated but those missing a leg or two are. Apart from humans, they're the only organisms known to do this.

Had I followed the route taken by my yoga ant as it exited my pants, I would have travelled deep into the rice fields of Bali to find its home. Wood ants live in large colonies, some with more than half a billion members in super-colonies containing a thousand interconnected nests. They survive cold winters in regions like the Swiss Jura mountains despite the frozen conditions. Their underground homes are kept warm by heat produced from rotting vegetation like a modern biomass central heating system.

But living in cramped conditions, surrounded by rot, infection can easily kill ants just as infection was trying to kill Ifan. How do ants thrive in such hostile conditions? Let's peer through the tiny doors to these big places where we will discover new drugs, new techniques of reducing antibiotic resistance and even ways to beat pandemics. Are you ready to live like an ant?

The first lesson of living like an ant is to tidy your bedroom. Ants are brilliant cleaners with dedicated waste-removal roles to ensure diseased items, like dead ants, are either removed from their nests or put in special sealed chambers. Like the Romans in their baths, ants have group cleaning rituals that help prevent disease. They groom themselves and others, even spraying acid on to individuals with evidence of infection on their bodies. Unlike my children, ants wash their hands before dinner. Had humans discovered this earlier, the lives of countless new mothers may have been saved.

Surprisingly, the link between handwashing and disease was made relatively recently. It was not until 1846 when a Hungarian doctor, Ignaz Semmelweis, started questioning why five times more women died of 'childbed fever' in hospital wards staffed by doctors compared with midwives.

Around this time, Semmelweis' pathology colleague pricked his finger while doing an autopsy on a young mother who had died from fever. Soon after, the pathologist too became sick and died. Semmelweis realised the pathologist had died from the same cause as the woman he had been examining. As it was only doctors who did autopsies, Semmelweis wondered if pieces of the dead on their hands were getting inside women during childbirth.

He ordered staff to clean their hands and instruments with a solution to help remove any smell from contact with infected tissue. As it happened, that solution was chlorine, still one of the most powerful antibacterials we have. As well as improving the smell, the chlorine washes dramatically reduced the numbers of graves that were being dug for mothers who had died in childbirth. The death rate plummeted in wards staffed by doctors, and Semmelweis had discovered handwashing, still one of public health's most important tools. Yet ants had been washing their hands for millions of years.

Now hospitals are strewn with antibacterial hand gel, with containers on most corners. I have even cared for patients in the intensive care unit who have become critically ill after drinking alcohol hand gel in desperation. Some modern hospitals also have robots that disinfect patient rooms using strong ultraviolet light. Yet even these modern, post-COVID norms have their roots in our ant ancestors.

Ants have long beaten humans to using UV light. In the hours after emerging from hibernation, ants swarm over the surface of their nests during sunny periods. They use the powerful solar UV rays to kill bacteria on the surface of their bodies after a long winter in cramped conditions being heated by rotting vegetation.

Wood ants also collect resin from spruce trees and place fragments in strategic locations around their underground home like hand gel in hospitals. This resin has been shown to kill pathogens including the antibiotic resistant bacteria MRSA. Humans are starting to learn from these techniques. South American indigenous peoples have long used the teeth of soldier ants to help stitch wounds, their antibiotic properties keeping wounds infection-free.

The oldest accounts of the therapeutic effects of coniferous resin stem from ancient Egypt, where soaps prepared from resin were used to treat burns. More recently, doctors in Finland have been testing tree resins on patients' wounds, showing they have antimicrobial, wound-healing and even skin regeneration-enhancing properties.

Ants then squirt formic acid, normally used to attack predators, on to the resin, sending an aerosol cloud of antibacterial particles into the air, spreading evenly throughout the nest. This disinfectant technique, using fogs, mists and aerosols, is now used in aeroplanes and for surface cleaning in operating theatres.

Some of the antibacterial fog will settle on the body of ants in the nest, much like we use antibacterial solutions to wash patients before major surgery to reduce the impact of skin-acquired infections.

But sometimes, UV and antiseptic just aren't enough. Although we had tried to keep Ifan's plastic lines into his body clean and to disinfect his skin, he still developed a severe infection. Despite the prevention strategies used in ants, they too can develop infections. But more significant for ant colonies is when their own food source develops an infection, because ants survive thanks to their love for mushrooms.

Fungus gardening ants have great skills in horticulture or, more correctly, fungiculture. You may have seen these ants carrying grass pieces, weighing hundreds of times their own weight, through your lawn towards their nests. These grass cuttings are used to nurture a fungus from the same family as the common button mushroom. It is this, not the grass directly, that the ants eat. Yet in these underground farms rages a viscous war of fungus vs fungus. The ants' fungus food is constantly attacked by a different type of microfungus in a fight to the death. Thankfully, ants have a powerful ally in this war, a friend with a special relationship who lives on their chests.

Bacteria from the Actinobacteria family are carried to faraway lands and protected by living on ants' bodies. Worker ants even coat eggs with these bacteria to form a lifelong relationship from the day an ant comes to life. As an ant matures, it feeds these bacteria nutrient-rich secretions from glands on its chest. The bacteria pay back the ants for this special care by making powerful antimicrobials that kill the microfungus that threatens its food gardens.

Researchers are finding large numbers of new antibiotic compounds from these Actinobacteria. These new drugs are active against very resistant human bacteria including

MRSA and fungi. Fungal infections, although less common than bacterial ones in humans, are a top cause of death in patients receiving immune treatments for cancer or living with an organ transplant. One of the most common fungi causing death in these patients is aspergillosis, killing as many as 90 per cent of patients who have this severe infection. Actinobacteria produce a number of agents likely to help in our fight against aspergillosis. One new drug called amycomicin is a very promising potent and specific antibiotic. In addition to fighting infections, investigating these compounds is important for anti-cancer and immune drug development. In fact, some chemotherapy drugs were originally developed as antifungals, including the drug sirolimus, found in soil Actinobacteria species on Easter Island. This now forms a cornerstone of care for patients having a kidney transplant.

The fact that bacteria make antibiotics is not really that surprising. Many drugs I prescribe were discovered from soil and ultimately made by microbes. What is crazily surprising, however, is that ant antibiotics still work so well after 100 million years of use. The microfungi that eat the ants' food should have evolved defences by now, yet ants still manage to keep infections at bay. When a new antibiotic drug is announced in human medicine, it is a predictably short period of time before the first bacteria to show resistance to it is identified. So how have ants kept effectiveness levels so high? What can we learn to aid human medicine? How can it help us treat Ifan?

One important strategy used by the bacteria on ants is to combine multiple types of antibiotic. They mix several kinds together into a marvellous medicine, using each for only short periods before changing their recipe, like a new brand of celebrity perfume that comes out every Christmas, subtly different to the last. The bacteria also share beneficial changes to their compounds that naturally occur through genetic shuffling with neighbouring bacteria. Like a deadly Rubik's Cube, they swap only new varieties with other bacteria that enhance killing of their enemies around them and keep them ahead of the game.

Recent discoveries from human trials have shown that mixing antibiotics prevents emergence of antibiotic resistance. The old teaching to always finish a course of antibiotics was ironically encouraging resistance to occur. Rather, short, sharp courses, rotating antibiotics from one to another, and using mixtures, just like ants, will help us protect future generations from a world where antibiotics are no longer effective.

And so, as Ifan's temperature burned, we rotated his antibiotics to one discovered from soil bacteria like that used in ants. We added others to his special mixture that would work together and be more than the sum of their parts. We used antiseptics in his mouth and on his wounds like the ants' resin in their underground nests. And as an improvement was seen, we stopped rather than continue his antibiotics to prevent resistance developing. We copied the ants at our feet, hoping that Ifan, like them, was strong enough to carry more than his body weight of critical illness and get through the dark times to see the sun's UV light rise again.

I had just spoken with Ifan's mum and dad, trying to arrange a good time to meet, when everything changed.

Everything.

Everything for me. For you. And for everyone.

On Tuesday, 10 March 2020, I packed my car with a sleeping bag, roll mat, food, toothpaste and clothes. I drove to the intensive care unit where I worked. I wasn't sure when I was going to be home again. I switched off my normal news radio station and put on something more relaxing – Mellow Magic.

I had upset my wife the evening before by sending her an email entitled 'Things you should know in case I die'. Along with computer passwords and the location of important documents, I had written:

'I've had a bloody wonderful life, travelled, partied, had two amazing children, spent time with friends, family, and done things I never dreamed of. I love my job even though it can be hard and dangerous. Touching the lives of others is the best feeling in the world.'

As I tried to start my standard thirteen-hour shift in intensive care, I didn't even know where to go. The hospital had been turned upside down and inside out. There were intensive care beds scattered where they were never meant to be.

That day, I cared for our hospital's first critically ill patient with COVID-19. We put him on to a life support machine, through the fogged plastic of a visor hastily put on before his oxygen plummeted so low that he could die. A week later there would be thirty such patients, then forty, then fifty. They didn't stop coming for over a year. As I write this, we are still caring for patients with COVID-19 in our intensive care unit.

Days earlier, my Canadian friend had sent me a photo showing how a hand sanitiser dispenser had been ripped off the wall at his hospital. My lunch that day was a cookie. For months, my wife said I was just a body with a phone attached. I tried to do bath and bed for my girls at night, but my mind was elsewhere. I slept in the spare room for months because I was always surrounded by viruses.

The best advice I was given early in the pandemic was no matter how busy you are, make sure you sit down and eat your lunch at a table – with a knife and fork. Like a human. None of this sandwich-on-the-go nonsense. It was great advice, that I couldn't take. Things were just too tough, too much. Much too much.

How did it feel to work in intensive care during a deadly viral pandemic? Unsurprisingly, the number of appropriate analogies is small. In the early days it felt a bit I imagine like being a first-time parent, living in a one-bedroom flat, when your baby came a month early, and that baby was one of triplets. You started parenthood feeling knackered after weeks of sleepless nights even before the babies arrived. Your good intentions to paint the nursery and have your bags packed slipped by. You worried about your ability to care for more children than you could hold. You also worried how you were going to get through unscathed. Even if you had enough cots and nappies, the physical infrastructure of your flat was not fit for purpose.

But we did get through it. Adrenaline, love, teamwork and hope were our fuel. The early days were hard, the later days even harder. I cried but I also laughed out loud. Did I come through unscathed? No. But most of the scars cannot be seen and they remind me of what was achieved. Life will never be the same again. Some parts worse, many parts, hopefully, eventually better.

In that time, I had put this book to one side. I cared for patients, saw them live, saw too many die, spoke on the TV and radio. I tried to give hope to the public, to give answers based on truth when I could and be honest by saying 'I don't know' when I did not.

I stopped reading about animals, I stopped reading about ants. This chapter was left half written, with Ifan's life hanging by a thread. And then, a year later, when the seas were calmer but the pubs still closed, I started again. And how I wished that I had kept reading about ants a year before. Because ants may have been able to save the world from some of the pain. Ants know how to deal with COVID-19.

They have known for 100 million years. And Dr Nathalie Stroeymeyt tried to tell us all of this years ago. Only now are we listening.

Nathalie's childhood wasn't unusual. Her mum was a teacher, her dad worked for a bank. They had a cat and moved from Belgium to a small village near Lille in the north of France when she was ten. A decade later, Nathalie spent a month gluing tiny QR codes on to the backs of more than 5,000 ants. And by doing so, she may have helped save the world from another deadly viral pandemic without even knowing it.

Speaking to her by videoconference in spring 2021, she had chosen the icing sugar-dusted Swiss mountains as her background. Walnut eyes, red cheeks and brown hair tied back, she seemed delicate, thoughtful, shy even. But the moment she started speaking about her ants, that all changed. Her hands moved with purpose, she spoke with confidence, insight and passion.

'Ants have already taught us so much,' she said with a half-smile. 'From theories of self-organisation, swarm intelligence, robotics, even how to best manage traffic jams. And now, perhaps, how to manage pandemics.'

It was a chance encounter with a French novel about a semi-fictionalised ant empire when she was a teenager that sparked her interest in what lies beneath our feet. After studying in university how ants manage conflict, ants took

Nathalie on a tour around research groups across Europe, from Paris to Copenhagen to Lausanne. Eventually, a $1.5 million research grant allowed her to set up her own ant behaviour lab in Bristol, England.

Her 2018 paper in the journal *Science*, 'Social network plasticity decreases disease transmission in a eusocial insect', was rated as one of the best research studies published that year. And it was all about how the behaviour of those 5,000 ants she had carefully labelled using Blu Tack on the end of matchsticks changed when infection hit their colony. Had it been read by government scientific advisers before the COVID-19 pandemic, I may have had a lot fewer families to break bad news to. A lot fewer hands that I needed to hold.

Nathalie is clear in pointing out that we cannot, and must not, make simple inferences from ants to humans. Ants have been balancing the risks and benefits from the measures they use for millions of years. Unlike humans, who have had extreme social isolation imposed without such time to adapt, we cannot say that what is best for ants is best for us, even if it is best for reducing disease. However, we can and should use lessons from ants as hints towards what is possible and effective.

Ants are remarkable not necessarily because of their characteristics as individuals. They cannot compete with the extraordinary heights of the Kenyan giraffe or the cuteness of a Western Australian koala. Instead, the beauty of ants lies in how they behave as a group, a community, a world.

Unlike humans, ants do not commonly die from disease. They die from severe trauma (being stood on) or catastrophic environmental damage (a raindrop). Although their resilience to infection, thanks to antimicrobials and antibiotics, may partially explain this, Nathalie thought that their behaviour must also play an important part. And she was right.

We now know ants specialise in not only their jobs, but in who they interact with. Only certain ants interact with high-value individuals like the queen, to reduce the chance of infections being transmitted. Ants shield the vulnerable.

Although grooming others helps prevent a build-up of infection, this close contact also has other advantages. It showers non-infected individuals with low-level exposure of bacteria allowing an immune response to form. Ants use a form of vaccination.

Individuals with low-level exposure even purposely contact others, resulting in transmission of this immunity. That is like vaccinated humans kissing someone to pass on the benefits of that vaccine indirectly.

If, despite these measures, a disease outbreak occurs, life quickly changes. Travel around the colony is severely restricted and social interaction plummets. Yes, ants socially distance.

Contacts are particularly reduced between those most vulnerable or valuable to the colony such as the queen, who becomes almost totally isolated physically and socially.

If an outbreak becomes even more serious, the colony's young, who are often a prime route of disease transmission as they are unable to move around, are removed from the nurturing environments where they normally develop, or are even murdered. This is not because they are more at risk from the disease themselves, but rather because the young cannot move and hence remain sites of infection to the wider colony. Although modern humans do not kill children to reduce disease transmission, we do remove them from places that encourage disease transmission like schools and childcare. And we too do this despite the direct risks to the children being low, in order to temper disease spread to the wider population. Ants seemingly close their schools.

And so, in pandemics, ants socially distance. They wash their hands. They protect the vulnerable and even form social bubbles in which interactions are restricted. They close their schools and use techniques that induce immunity. Ants have a system of public health that we have just developed.

And sadly, ants also behave in death as so many were forced to do with COVID-19. Ants not only live altruistically, but they also die altruistically. Ants who are dying abandon their nests to die in seclusion, reducing the risk of transmitting disease to close relatives.

Over the last year, regrettably, I have held the hands of many patients who have died without their families being there. Distance was needed for safety, yet distance compounds sadness. I'll forever remember the songs that mothers and fathers and sons and daughters asked me to play as someone they loved died when they could not be there. It was a playlist for the pandemic that I never wanted to hear. Perhaps, just perhaps, if we had looked at the way that some of our ant ancestors deal with infection, this playlist could have been a lot shorter.

We started our exploration of land animals before the beginning, before birth. We saw how kangaroos helped humans nurture life, first inside the body and then outside, after the birth of the world's first test-tube baby, Louise Brown. The touch of our orangutan past helped care for Lucy's premature triplets through the glare of their glass incubators. The koala helped us understand our inner microbiome world. We now know that what comes out of our bodies is as important as what goes in. Finally, we met Ifan, bleeding on to the pavement but helped to his feet by the brain and breathing of the mighty African giraffe. But just as we needed to begin at the beginning, we need to end at the end.

After weeks in the intensive care unit, countless bad news conversations with his mum and dad, Ifan's struggle did end. His brain started to calm. His infection relented. Ifan's eyes opened to a sunny Welsh February morning, as another journey began. His recovery would be long, with ups and downs. Life would not be the same again. Just like after COVID-19, many parts different, some worse, some parts, eventually, better.

In the distance, I could see Ifan sitting on the side of a rugby pitch in the park with his mum and enjoying the summer's day. Finally, we could meet again. Shaved head, big scar, shorts and a T-shirt with his favourite Welsh band on the front. His handshake felt good. Strong. I told him about giraffes and ants. He smiled, he laughed, he reminisced and said thank you to the mystery man who had given him first aid on that blooded street after being assaulted. He showed me his jumper, made by a company he has started. On the front is written the Welsh word 'Wyddfa', the Celtic name for Wales's highest mountain. Meaning 'grave', it is believed that the giant Rhita Gawr was buried in the rocky cliffs known as Snowdon in English.

Ifan was far from the grave now. He said life was strangely clearer than before. He could see more of what was always there. Everything was more vibrant, more beautiful, even the rot. I guess being so close to death can do that to you.

I said that a hundred lifetimes wouldn't suffice to see all the beauty in one acre of land. He smiled and nodded as he waved away a flying ant from his face into the air above.

THE AIR

'Like petals in the wind, we're puppets to the silver strings of souls, of changes.'

PHIL OCHS

6

LIGHTING UP THE DARK

Two men float into darkness. A flimsy boat made from flax stems bobs, struggling to hold their weight. They come from different places, different cultures, different worlds. Tane Tinorau, New Zealand's Kāwhia tribe's Māori chief. A powerful tree of a man, long black beard, deep eyes, knowing. He found the cave's small entrance guarded by a den of wild dogs a few years earlier. Lying, body against body, alongside him holding a wax candle is Fred Mace. An English surveyor, rounded glasses, oversized moustache, receding hairline, pale. These unlikely friends from worlds apart are passengers on the underground blackwater stream running deep into an undiscovered cave. They aren't nervous but tiptoeing on the edge of comfort, as amateur explorers did in 1888.

Pushing deeper underground using a pole made from a tall native kauri tree, they enter a cathedral cave the height of a six-storey building. Water drops fall from stalactites, echoing. As the candle flickers, high above and all around shines the light from a million blue stars. Yet these are not stars.

The explorers stretch back in their raft, lying down to look high at the glowing celling. The candle is blown out. They stare upwards, say nothing, wonder at what makes this cave come alive with light. The neon blue glow dapples on the black water around the boat. They had discovered Waitomo Caves, Māori for waterhole, in New Zealand's North Island.

More than 100 years later, I travelled to Waitomo. I retraced the ripples made by the explorers in a much sturdier boat, armed with the knowledge of what makes the caves glow. I too stretched backwards, lay on my raft, switched off my head torch and stared up. There were still millions of blue stars, the glow of chemical fire made by Arachnocampa luminosa, a fungal gnat native to New Zealand, commonly called a glow-worm. Breaking down its luciferin compound with the luciferase enzyme creates a glow known as bioluminescence.

The same bioluminescence surrounded cancer patient Bill Ludwig as he sat on his New Jersey porch one night that same summer I went to New Zealand. While fireflies danced, he wondered if he would live or die. If beating his cancer were possible, it was thanks to the glow around him.

In the summer of 2000, I emerged from that black water cave in New Zealand, helped by the descendants of Tane Tinorau who still work there. My hands and feet were so cold that hot water from the shower afterwards felt like frozen hailstones piercing my skin. While I was recovering from the shock and awe of the glow-worms, on the other side of the world in New Jersey, 54-year-old Bill Ludwig was recovering from his own life-changing moment. After having what should have been a simple hernia repair, he left hospital with a terminal condition. A routine test done before his operation found blood cancer – chronic lymphocytic leukaemia.

Bill vowed to fight on as he had fought throughout his life. Entering the US Marine Corps in 1962 straight from high school, he helped blockade Cuba during the nuclear missile crisis. His 10th artillery division, nicknamed the 'Arm of Decision', had the motto 'King of Battle'. This tactic of blockade rather than declaration of war likely saved us all from a terrible nuclear fate.

By the time Bill's chemotherapy started, he was working at Bayside State Prison as a correction officer. It was a modern institution where inmates did meaningful work in the prison's dairy. It was also a busy prison with more than 2,000 inmates, half guilty of violent crimes.

One notorious inmate was George Wright. During a thirty-year sentence for murder, he escaped, driving a prison warden's car to the airport before hijacking Delta Air Lines flight 841 dressed as a priest, along with four others. After a $1 million ransom was paid, the hijackers took the plane to Algeria, where they escaped.

'He'd do chemo and go to work the same day,' Bill's wife recalled. 'He just felt he had a job to do, and did it.'

In 2007, Bill retired after becoming increasingly

debilitated. The chemotherapy kept his leukaemia at bay but took a toll on his ageing body. The cancer always remained with him, grumbling through the veins under his skin, in his organs and his bone marrow.

'We knew he was going to die,' his wife said. 'Then Alison told him about the clinical trial.'

Alison is actually Professor Alison Loren, the head of bone marrow transplant at the University of Pennsylvania's world-leading hospital. She told me when we first met that 'blood is beautiful'. It had long fascinated her: the colour, the texture, its functions, the way it flows, the way it dries. When she was just five, her next-door neighbour, a sweet girl around nine years old, died of leukaemia. Later, at medical school, she thought about that little girl when looking down a microscope at the blood cells that had killed her. She was determined to make a difference and what a difference she did make. Today, her next-door neighbour would survive her leukaemia with the modern treatment regimens developed by Professor Loren and her colleagues. But even these were not enough for Bill.

It takes around fifteen years and more than $1 billion to move a cancer drug from the theoretical laboratory into the first patient. The explosion in genetic research over the past fifty years promised to reduce these costs and has coloured our understanding of many diseases that cause death and suffering. The discovery of genes that switch cancer pathways on and off in our bodies transformed the 'Big C' from a lifestyle to a genetic disease. However, in the next fifty years, cancer will be better understood as a problem with our immune system as well as our genes.

Even after medical school, my understanding of our immune system was limited to 'white blood cells'. Yet inside us all is an astonishingly complex system, more intertwined and connected than large modern cities. Hundreds of different cell types with different jobs, talking with your tissues and hormones and proteins even while you sleep. Whispers from your lungs are heard by blood vessels in your kidneys. These conversations release just the right chemicals at just the right times.

All this aims to not only keep infectious invaders at bay, but to weed out errors made by our own cellular factories that churn out new cells from a genetic blueprint every second of every day. When any cell replicates, the shuffling nature of genetics introduces random errors. While most mistakes are irrelevant and would go unnoticed, key changes in genes controlling replication could make cells multiply uncontrollably. Cancer results. And so our immune system spots these errors, hunts down rogue cells and destroys them before a cancer army can be formed.

In Bill's case, his immune B-cells that normally produce antibodies had gone rogue. Genetic errors were not spotted and they were replicating out of control. Over 3kg of cancer cells were raging though Bill's bloodstream and living in his bone marrow. The chemotherapy was a blunt hammer, killing all cells that were dividing. That included healthy cells, meaning that each cycle of treatment made Bill's body weaker while only killing a small percentage of his cancer cells.

Through understanding the importance of the immune system in cancer development, researchers imagined new ways to treat cancers like Bill's. Could they engineer immune cells to hunt down Bill's own rogue B-cells? This would allow only cancer cells to be targeted and selectively killed. They called this technique chimeric antigen receptor T-cell therapy (CART-T). It was a brilliant idea. But researchers would need to look inside living cells, in real time, to make it work. These tools didn't exist.

The genetic revolution had been made possible thanks to new discoveries like the polymerase chain reaction (PCR) that allowed rapid copying and analysis of genetic code. Then specialised enzymes were developed, allowing the codes that make individual genes to be broken apart and glued back together. Today, modern techniques like CRISPR/Cas9 allow far more detailed, inexpensive genetic engineering. DNA sequences can be quickly and cheaply altered letter by letter, modifying gene function, correcting medical defects or even improving the growth and resilience of crops.

Yet despite powerful tools at a genetic level, researchers struggled to study the proteins that are made by genes in living tissues. Experiments would instead need to kill animal models, stain their tissues with dyes and wait days or weeks after treatments to see what was happening inside. With only such basic tools, many advances in cancer treatments like that to be trialled in Bill would simply not have been possible.

What humanity needed was ways to track, in real time, changes to proteins that genetic manipulation could make. Cancer should be studied in life, not in thin slices of death seen down a microscope. And all this should be possible without altering the underlying functions of the cells being studied. Who would have thought this puzzle could be solved by fireflies, glow-worms and jellyfish?

The answers came from 'unforeseen events and circumstances, scientific study, people, and chances that led to unimagined results'. These are the words of Osamu Shimomura, a Japanese scientist who won a Nobel Prize for showing how mysterious animals glow with brilliant light in deep oceans and dark nights. It was this unlikely discovery that allowed cancer cures like those tested in Bill to be possible. But first, Osamu Shimomura needed to survive a nuclear war.

The first day of middle school for sixteen-year-old Osamu Shimomura was not as he expected. It was 1945 and the Second World War raged on in Japan, where he lived. His mathematics lesson was abandoned as the headmaster told students they were being sent to a fighter plane repair factory instead of doing trigonometry. The battered single-seater Japanese Mitsubishi 'Zero' planes kept coming until, two months later, the factory stood empty. A move to the suicidal kamikaze tactic, where pilots would plunge into the sides of ships, killing themselves in the process, meant that few planes returned.

On 9 August 1945, the all-too familiar wailing of the air raid siren sounded across the factory floor where Osamu now worked. After the all-clear was given at 8.30 a.m., rather than return to work, Osamu and his friends climbed a nearby hill and watched a sole American B-29 bomber glide across the sky. It was assumed to be a reconnaissance plane and no further alarm sounded. Three soft white parachutes fell gently to the ground from the plane. American soldiers, perhaps? Another B-29 came into view. Then the world changed.

A blinding flash, pressure waves shattered factory windows, a downpour of black, sticky rain poured on to Osamu's silk shirt, which his grandma had made from silkworms in her garden. Panic, debris, the air tasted different. Buildings fell. People, animals and clocks all died. Then silence.

Osamu witnessed the 'Fat Man' bomb being dropped on Nagasaki, the largest nuclear explosion in history, killing 70,000 people almost instantly. It consumed hospitals, homes, the medical school and sacred spaces such as the Sanno Shinto Shrine and the Urakami Cathedral. After running home covered in dust like a ghost in the fog, his grandmother took off the sticky black shirt and bathed Osamu, unknowingly saving his life from radiation sickness. Nagasaki was destroyed. Osamu lived. He wasn't special, but lucky.

Through the devastation, life did go on. Hours turned to days and days to years. Although Osamu had little interest in the subject, joining a rebuilt pharmacy school was his only chance of an education. He graduated top of his class and stumbled through jobs and teaching positions as Nagasaki was slowly put back together again. Osamu hoped a meeting with a top university biologist would change his fortune. Osamu arrived at the professor's office, only to find he was away for the day. Deflated, walking down the corridor, he started talking to an organic chemist with a strange obsession with a crustacean called the Japanese sea-firefly.

'Come to my lab. You can start any time,' he said to Osamu.

And so he did.

By 1961, Osamu had already significantly advanced the understanding of bioluminescence through his research. A year earlier, the newly married Osamu had sailed for thirteen days on an old hospital boat from Japan to the US for a fellowship at Princeton. Battling death threats and racial prejudice, his experiments moved on from studying just the sea-firefly.

Osamu had already shown that glowing creatures, like the sea-firefly, emit blue light when compounds called luciferin (Latin for light-bearer) were broken down by enzymes called luciferase. Osamu became the first person to purify luciferin and crystallise it using strong acids. This allowed its structure to be studied and understood. At the time, it was thought that the light of all bioluminescent organisms was produced by this luciferin/luciferase reaction. But the glowing ring of light around the crystal jellyfish he had seen in Princeton seemed different. Although jellyfish can be thought of as just organised water, some species also glow like fireflies. But Osamu had a hunch that a different mechanism may be responsible.

In 1965, not long after Bill Ludwig was helping prevent another nuclear war in Cuba, Osamu was in the Waitomo Caves staring at those same glow-worms on the celling. He thought back to stories his dad had told of Japanese soldiers using dried sea-fireflies to read maps by their dim blue light. Although he would miss Japan, during that trip Osamu decided to make Princeton his permanent home. There he would be best placed to solve the mystery of the glowing jellyfish.

To do this, every summer Osamu would drive 3,000 miles across the US to a sleepy seaside village called Friday Harbor on the west coast. There his young family would spend the early morning hours walking around the docks netting jellyfish. One summer, they collected over forty buckets a day until 10,000 jellyfish had been caught. This allowed his team to purify just 1mg of the mysterious glowing chemical. Yet all of Osamu's efforts to purify a new luciferin-like compound failed.

Late one evening, Osamu threw yet another failed experiment down the sink. As the macerated tissue hit the porcelain with a slap, a nuclear glow rose from the white sink. The room was lit by vivid green–blue light. His mind raced, rapid further experiments late into the night showed the seawater from an old fish tank draining into the sink had somehow caused the jellyfish to glow. Days later, he had cracked it. It was the calcium in the seawater that turned transparent jellyfish flesh into a glowing beacon. But so what? Who would care?

Nearly fifty years later, a phone call at 5.15 a.m. told 80-year-old Osamu Shimomura that he had won the Nobel Prize. The frail Osamu stood on stage in Stockholm during the award ceremony, grey suit hanging off his squared shoulders, trembling hands. He stuttered to a start, recalling the blinding glow of the atomic bomb that, through the hand of serendipity, had led him to discover the green glow of life. His finding may have helped save even more than the 70,000 people killed that terrible nuclear day in Nagasaki.

Reaching into his jacket pocket, Osamu removed a small tube of liquid made from more than 20,000 jellyfish. Activating it with a small UV light, he held the now bright glowing green beacon high above his head. His hands were still shaking but he was transformed into a Japanese super-hero. His still face came to life as the audience clapped and smiled as the auditorium lights were dimmed and green shone all around.

Osamu had discovered green fluorescent protein, now known in laboratories all around the world simply as 'GFP'.

Over nineteen summers, his team collected 850,000 jelly-fish from Friday Harbor. The compound he found held the key to understanding fluorescence, illuminance and biolu-minescence, how it can be triggered and what species from the glow-worm in New Zealand caves to the firefly on Bill Ludwig's porch have in common.

But to understand why GFP allowed a revolution in cancer treatments we need to meet another scientist. As Osamu was collecting jellyfish in 1965 and Bill Ludwig was keeping the peace by sea in Cuba, Martin Chalfie was also surrounded by water as the captain of Harvard's swim team. He would become one of the two other scientists to share the stage with Osamu during the 2008 Nobel Prize cere-mony. They helped transform an interesting green glowing protein into an essential tool for the study of cancer.

Seventy-three years old, blue T-shirt, greyed moustache stretching across the width of his face. Tinted glasses, sitting in front of bright floor-to-ceiling windows, shuffling in his chair, sitting on his hands, talking to me from Vermont. Martin Chalfie is still in love with science.

The summer after his junior year in college, he failed at every experiment he did. He felt like a failure. He would never be a scientist, he thought. During his senior year, Chalfie spent more time thinking about drama and Dostoevsky than science.

Separated from friends and family at Harvard in 1965, he

told me he felt 'at sea'. And so, ironically, he threw himself into swimming as a way to make friends and connect with people who had common interests. It made him feel like himself again. He was good at it too, soon becoming captain of the swim team between 1968 and 1969. As Chalfie swam up and down the lanes, 3,000 miles away, the width of the country, thousands of jellyfish were being caught by Osamu, who really was at sea.

Although GFP was discovered in 1962, it took nearly thirty years for its practical applications to become clear. Chalfie did become a scientist despite his tricky start that first summer. He specialised in how worms sense the world around through touch. After listening to a talk on bioluminescence by chance, Chalfie wondered if the green glowing marker could help him track genetic changes in his own experiments with worms.

Despite having no funding for the idea, Chalfie's group successfully integrated GFP into a single gene inside E. coli bacteria. They hoped GFP could help keep track of which genes became activated by shining light on to bugs while still alive. It worked. A photo of a Petri dish, half glowing green, soon appeared in major scientific journals. A third scientist, Roger Tsien, extended the experiments, genetically manipulating GFP to make it brighter and shine all the colours of the rainbow. Finally, the tools were ready. Treatments like chimeric antigen receptor T-cell therapy (CART-T) could be tried and tested.

Chalfie's phone, like those of Osamu and Tsien, rang in 2008 to tell him of his Nobel Prize. The old landline in his

New York apartment kitchen kept ringing out behind two thick closed doors. Chalfie slept through the best news of his life. Research in fields as strange as fireflies, jellyfish and worms can lead to astounding things. Just sometimes they can help cure cancer.

'All life should be studied,' says Chalfie.

'Not just as models, but as life itself.'

The colourful glow from GFP revolutionised experimental cancer science. It led slowly but surely to these advanced treatments like CART-T. Scientists now had the tools to test and track advanced genetic changes like sticking new protein receptors on the surface of immune cells. They could now do this in living tissue, in real time, and hopefully with real-world results.

Scientists soon used GFP technology to track a virus infecting immune T-cells. They could see in glowing green that a new protein receptor had successfully been added to the surface of the immune cells. They watched these new mutant cells hunt down and kill rogue cancer cells yet leave healthy cells untouched. CART-T worked. In a dish. But would it work in person? Bill was willing to find out.

On his wedding anniversary in July 2008, the cancer team at Penn University started Bill's treatment. A needle in his arm sucked blood towards a machine that spun around 5,000 times per minute. This separated the emulsion of cells in Bill's thick cancerous blood. The white blood cells were guided into a plastic bag before being carefully carried down a corridor to be further separated. His precious T-cells were then deliberately infected with a harmless virus, which added a new gene to the cell's DNA. This new copy-and-pasted gene made a specially designed protein on the surface of Bill's own T-cells. It was this surface protein receptor that would recognise cancer cells.

Bill's new hacked T-cells grew in dishes, multiplying more than 700 times before being packaged and sent back to the clinic. Two weeks later, Bill returned to have these designer cells pushed back into his body through that same vein they had exited. The multiplication process continued more then 10,000 times but now inside him.

No one really knew what would happen. Bill was the first patient to have this treatment. Would the journey from Nagasaki, the death, the destruction, the glow of more than 850,000 jellyfish that led to the Nobel Prize save him?

'Did I ever think it would be successful?' Bill was asked. 'Not in a million years.'

7

Keeping cool

Days after the experimental treatment Bill was sick enough to die. This was bad, but also strangely good.

It was a summer's day in Pennsylvania but the Appalachian surroundings kept the temperature a comfortable 20°C. Yet, despite being surrounded by whirling fans and wide-open windows, Bill's body was burning up from the inside. His normal 37.5°C temperature fired to over 40°C as his nurse threw away thermometers, thinking they were broken. They weren't. Bill was. But he was also healing.

The new cancer treatment, made possible through fire-flies' glow, had turned Bill's own immune system into a cancer-killing machine. It was hard at work destroying the 3kg of cancerous blood cells in his body. But the assault had started to get out of control. He was soon taken to the intensive care unit, with all his major organs shutting down. The fluid that doctors squeezed into his veins to help his blood pressure was leaking out like water through a sieve. His legs swelled to twice their normal size. Doctors strug-gled to control his temperature. They would need to use a technology inspired by cold animal feet in frozen lakes.

Professor Loren picked up the phone to call Bill's wife, remembering the last words he had said to her – 'I trust you.'

'I don't think he's going to see the sunrise,' she said.

Medicine and life are all about balance. Finding that sweet spot, that equilibrium. We walk along the edge where the ocean meets the sand, sometimes moving into the sea to cool off, sometimes lying on the beach to glow hot. The treatment that was killing Bill's cancer was also killing him. It was out of equilibrium, rampaging away. We call this reaction hyperinflammation. The chemical signals in your blood go wild, your organs shut down and you can die. Sometimes caused by drugs, or infections, or CART-T, hyperinflammation is also seen with COVID-19.

My work caring for critically ill patients often involves letting patients cure themselves. We support the organs while bodies heal. This needs machines and nurses and drugs, but ultimately the real cure is often time. Sometimes, doing nothing is hard. There is a temptation to intervene, to add, to fiddle. So I remind myself: 'Don't just do something – stand there!' This is not the case with hyperinflammation. Without the right treatment, quickly, the body can consume itself. When we treat patients like Bill today, we do two things quickly – control the temperature and stop the fire.

Our fire extinguisher is a drug that acts like a key chemical in the body, the master controller of our body's inflammatory system. This substance is so important that it dates back to the world's earliest animal – 558 million years old. The chemical even helped prove an ancient fossil was actually an animal and not a plant. Sadly, Bill's illness occurred before doctors knew about the potential of this drug. So they were left desperately trying to cool his body. They found inspiration from animals that constantly battle with extremes of temperature. I headed to the frozen fields of Canada's north to meet that animal, the whooping crane.

I left the Maple Leaf Lounge at London's Heathrow Airport having eaten maple leaf-shaped waffles for breakfast, washed down with a cold Canadian beer. The flight went over Iceland, skirted the frozen coast of Greenland, before descending into Vancouver. The short stopover was during the Super Bowl final, cheers and beer glasses clinking all around. Canadians seemed to be watching a game of rugby with helmets on while I tried to check the score for Wales playing the real game in the Six Nations tournament. Two countries separated by a common sport, perhaps?

A connecting flight took me to the frozen lands of Alberta. The view from the plane as we approached the runway to land was a terrifying descent into a sheer white surface that looked more like an ironed tablecloth than an airport. Yet the pilot headed down to the snow, landing the plane with a squeak and a skid. The taxi ride from the airport was even more exhilarating, any semblance of road markings covered by snow and ice. I started to understand why Canada had legalised marijuana. It was a warm winter day for Alberta, just twenty under. I spent my first week with a Canadian doctor who had become a friend through shared writing, shared experiences and shared conference stages. He took me skiing for the first time, where I failed to graduate from the Penguin starter class after being shown up by children barely old enough to walk. The ice skating (falling) at -25°C was a tough day for my fingers and now blue toes, but the company, the beauty of the country and the hot coffee kept me going.

But I hadn't come all this way for Starbucks. I had come to meet a bird found in the remote wilderness of the Canadian northlands that laughs in the face of low temperatures. Even without the latest Gore-Tex merino wool, the whooping crane stands for hours feeding in glacial frozen lakes, without its toes turning blue. Understanding how would help doctors cool patients like Bill and many others with rocketing temperatures.

The journey into the wilderness was long and brutal. Snow everywhere. Ice everywhere. Miles measured in hundreds not tens. But finally, a glimpse. Snow-white, stick-black bony legs, flash of red on the head. Quiet. Still. Standing in a frozen lake. Black-tipped wings set off against the snow backdrop. Tall. Over 1.5 metres. Then – a twig snaps under my foot, the crane's head cranks up and a shriek-like trumpet call goes out. The sound travels far, over a kilometre, warning others of my twig snap. But it isn't the whooping sound produced that makes this animal so significant. It is the long slender legs at the opposite end of its body that will help control Bill's temperature.

Whooping cranes spend winter in Aransas near the Texas Gulf Coast. For decades, no one knew where they flew to each spring to breed other than 'north'. Then, in 1954, a wildfire broke out in a remote part of Canada's Wood Buffalo National Park. Firefighters spotted two large white birds, later confirmed by the biologist, W. A. Fuller, to be whooping cranes from the last remaining wild population. The park, which had been created in 1922 to safeguard wood bison, became critical for another species at risk. There are now more than 500 of the world's 826 whooping cranes in Wood Buffalo National Park in Alberta.

At the end of many beds in my intensive care unit sits a big grey machine. It looks like a photocopier but with blue pipes running out from its base towards the patient lying on the bed. A bright digital screen dances with colourful lines draw-ing a continuous line graph. Following the blue pipes towards the patient, they connect to large sticky blue pads wrapped around the body like clingfilm around a sandwich. And run-ning through plastic veins inside these pads is ice cold water, cooling down patients as it runs across their skin. Sucking away heat generated from inflammation, the machine targets a sweet spot of not too hot, not too cold. Just right.

This way of cooling critically ill patients uses the same method as the whooping crane I was watching in the Canadian wilderness. As the bird stood in a frozen lake, its feet should freeze solid. Frostbite should set in and the bird should die. Yet it didn't, thanks to a system of central heating pipework.

Each vein in the bird's thin legs carries blood from deep underwater up towards the heart. These veins travel in parallel to arteries carrying warm blood from deep inside the body. Running in opposite directions, right next to each other, the blood vessels form a counter-current heat exchange system that minimises heat loss. Warm arteries transfer heat to the cold veins, allowing birds to feed in ice cold lakes without losing their legs. Then, in hotter summer months, this process is reversed, distributing heat from arteries into the cooler veins that dive down into cold water.

This is just like the complex network of plastic channels in the cooling devices used in intensive care. Using a cold water reservoir in the machine instead of a glacial Canadian lake, water would flow continually over Bill's burning body under the plastic pads. Bill's veins would cool down after heat is sucked out, returning to his heart to cool the rest of his body. The higher the flow rates of water, the more cooling; the colder the water temperature, the more cooling. And when treating hypothermic patients pulled from the sea, this principle is reversed like a crane in the lake, to bring their body temperature slowly back to normal.

Even without a global viral pandemic ruining travel plans, there is one animal species that helps us cool patients that I could never meet. Despite being at the top of the food chain, for the 5-tonne and 13-metre-long largest land carnivore, the biggest challenge was staying cool. Eighty million years ago, the Tyrannosaurus rex came up with a novel plan still used today.

For years, two large gaps at the back of its fossilised head were thought to be filled with powerful jaw muscles. These holes, also found in crocodiles and lizards, evolved about 300 million years ago. Thermal imaging studies in modern animals have shown these holes light up on cold days, turn off on warm days. It is now known that instead of muscles, they were filled with blood vessels used to heat the brain when cold and cool it down when hot. The Tyrannosaurus rex had an air conditioning system for its brain.

These techniques are now used in the RhinoChill system, a medical device that provides emergency brain cooling. A tube delivers a mist of perfluorohexane coolant up a patient's nose. This evaporates after contact with the nasal cavity acting as a rapid heat exchanger, cooling the base of the skull and the brain. For some patients who have a cardiac arrest, this Tyrannosaurus rex-style brain cooling can reduce the chances of brain damage by almost a third, preventing their extinction.

Cooling Bill's body didn't address the root cause of his illness. It was the cellular chaos that was killing his body. But there is a treatment that could have stopped it. The same chemical that could turn down the heat had been used by the world's oldest animals to survive. The drug had been discovered over seventy years ago.

The American chemist Luis Fieser holds a contrary place in history. On the one hand he was instrumental in producing a drug that has saved the lives of countless people. On the other, he also invented a weapon that led to the needless suffering of countless others. Fieser synthesised the steroid drug cortisone, alongside others including vitamin K. But he also discovered the sticky, firebomb chemical napalm. Shortly after the bombing of Nagasaki that eventually led to the technology behind Bill's cancer treatment, Fieser's napalm would kill many more Japanese than atom bombs. But his steroid drugs could help cure hyperinflammation and even COVID-19.

We commonly associate steroids with muscle-clad bodybuilders or disgraced athletes using them as performance-enhancing drugs. However, they are a broad class of chemicals found in all complex creatures. Steroids act as chemical signallers, telling different tissues to grow, shrink, release chemicals or even go to sleep. Steroids also dampen down inflammation, a firehose against the heat of disease.

In June 1948, a fifty-year-old farmer's wife could no longer even squeeze her washcloth, her joints were so red hot with rheumatoid arthritis. Every twenty-four hours felt like 'one more day of misery and pain is past'. Arriving by wheelchair at the Mayo Clinic in Rochester, Minnesota, for an experimental treatment, she was injected with 'compound E' made from ground cows' adrenal glands. Within a week she 'walked out of the hospital in a gay mood and went on a shopping trip'. The steroid chemicals in this cow juice had dampened down her joint inflammation.

Huge quantities of adrenal glands were needed to produce even tiny amounts of medicine – 50kg for just the 200mg of steroids used daily in many hospitalised patients today. Synthetic production was therefore critical and it was hoped more selective chemicals would also reduce the side effects, which included swelling from water retention, gastric acidity and psychosis.

With heightened interest in synthetic steroid hormone production for oral contraceptive use in the 1950s, Fieser led the industrial research. He perfected the production process and launched the drug cortisone in 1950. Steroids have remained the most widely prescribed medications in the world ever since. They are now key compounds that treat hyperinflammation due to CART-T therapy and dramatically reduce deaths by a third in patients critically ill with COVID-19. They saved an estimated 1 million people during the pandemic thanks to their low cost and global availability. Yet animals have long been trying to tell us of the importance of this key chemical. In 2021, as if to underline their significance even further, steroids helped identify the oldest animal on earth.[*]

---

[*]   Bobrovskiy, I. et al. Ancient steroids establish the Ediacaran fossil Dickinsonia as one of the earliest animals. Science **361**, 1246–1249 (2018).

Five hundred and fifty-eight million years ago, a 1.4-metre-long object fell gently to the bottom of the sea where the South Australian Flinders mountain ranges sit today. It didn't see daylight again until 1940 when a palaeontologist called Reginald Sprigg named it Dickinsonia after Ben Dickinson, the director of South Australia mines. Scientists have since debated whether Dickinsonia is a primitive animal, a bacterial colony or just a plant. Finally, in 2021, scientists discovered traces of steroids in the preserved fossil. This proved that the 558-million-year-old object was indeed the oldest animal ever found as these steroids are only found in life of this form. And this animal needed steroids to survive.

Seven days spent in the intensive care unit feels like an age for patients and their families. Bill's burning temperature was cooled after one week thanks to the whooping crane's technology but the powerful effects of the steroids would have to wait. His cancer treatment was so novel that Professor Loren's team thought the extreme heat and inflammation was due to infection rather than Bill's body attacking itself.

Today, I treat patients hot with hyperinflammation from CART-T early with steroids and the immune drug tocilizumab, which neutralises a powerful cytokine causing inflammation called IL-6. We do this thanks to the lessons learnt from pioneers like Professor Loren and Bill, who needed to use just time as a healer. Ironically, Bill would develop another new disease in the future, one that could also be treated with steroids and tocilizumab. But again, he would become ill too soon, before doctors realised these treatments could help.

Thankfully, with time alone, Bill's body did heal. The cooling machines were turned down and his racing heart slowed to a jog. Remarkably, his cancer was shrinking too. Seven days in ICU led to a month spent on a hospital ward. Bill was weak and skeletal. But was he cancer-free? Professor Loren ordered a bone marrow biopsy to check the level of cancer cells in Bill's blood. She thought about those words Bill had said to her – 'I trust you.' They weighed heavily as the results came through. What if Bill had been through all of this, had nearly died in a sterile ICU, for nothing?

A few days later, Professor Loren was frustrated and confused. Bill's results just didn't make sense. The lab must have mixed them up with someone else's. They couldn't have been right. They were far too good. A repeat sample of Bill's bone marrow was taken. There had not been a mix-up. The cancer had gone. Completely.

Ten years after Bill's cancer was treated, Professor Loren still looks at the postcards pinned to the wall in her office. Bill and his wife bought a motor home and didn't stop touring. They didn't just spend time drinking tea on folding chairs either. Life happens in the cracks, in the places between there and here. The in-between lands. The couple learnt to white water raft and ride horses. They romped with their dogs, Maddie and Fozzie. They walked on the sunny side of the street. And they celebrated holidays, births, graduations, weddings. Life returned. The cancer did not. Bill had put his trust in the right place.

8

SCRATCHING AN ITCH

It was a long way to go just to be bitten, naked – 500 miles, three countries, two bridges, a car ferry, a boat, a quad bike and an hour's walk. But it was worth it.

I have travelled to the bone-breakingly beautiful island of Eilean Shona in the West Scottish Highlands. A rugged and rocky 2 miles by 1 mile island. From the 850ft peak Beinn a'Bhaillidh, you can gaze to Rum, Eigg and Skye to the west and Ben Nevis to the east. The motorboat picked me up aside the ruins of Castle Tiora, built in the thirteenth century and where, 300 years later, Prince Charles held sway over western Scotland through loyal supporters of the Jacobite cause.

Middle-age stiffness set in from my twelve-hour drive from Cardiff, my right arm ridiculously tanned from its sunny window position. I survived the drive by listening to the 'Greatest Albums in the World' that I'd never listened to before – Bob Dylan's *Blood on the Tracks*, *The Dark Side of the Moon* from Pink Floyd and Joni Mitchell's *Blue*.

But my walk from the island jetty to my secluded Red Cottage was filled with the sounds of life, not music. A seal splashed in the mirrored waters, a herd of wild deer trampled over roots, an oversized white-tailed eagle straight from Jurassic Park circled above. Had I been secretly transported into a Disney movie?

The whole island looked dip-dyed in soft green velvet. The one large main house was founded by a Captain Swinburne as a hunting lodge in the nineteenth century. He developed the most diverse pine plantation in Europe, which now homes rare groups of pine martens collectively called a 'richness'.

I'm not the first writer to be lost in this island's magic. It is the original real-life Neverland. J. M. Barrie wrote Peter Pan here after writing to friends 'a wild rocky romantic island it is, too' and 'This is a very lovely spot, almost painfully so'.* My solitary week was spent with no cars, no Wi-Fi, no phone signal but ample single malt whisky. A massive storm soon took down the limited electricity meaning that writing was done by candlelight. Later that week, a two-hour hike up a mountain gave one bar of mobile signal, enough to tell my family I was alive. The three essential items for any walk included a coat, a camera and binoculars. The things you really didn't need were a key, as all the cottages remain unlocked, or a broken ankle.

I did things that I genuinely thought only happen in films – I drank from a river, foraged for food, walked with a big stick. A cold loch swim at dusk under a newly formed

---

* From a letter dated 13 August 1920, published in 1942 by Viola Meynell in a collection called 'Letters by JM Barrie'. Also quoted in an article titled 'Unlocking the magic of Eilean Shona' by Rosanna Dodds in the *Financial Times*, 10 December 2021.

rainbow after 'Polly's Power Hour', an exercise class held in a makeshift wooden town hall, reminded me to do what I had really come for.

Back at Red Cottage, a glug of whisky, my loch-soaked clothes in a puddle on the floor, my body bare. I opened the door to a quiet dusk, walked forwards between pine and fern and a red-topped wild mushroom. All around me, a cloud of dander flitted then landed on to skin. To feed. To bite. I had come for the midges; the midges had come for me.

I was told a story about a Scottish schoolteacher who had quit his job to embark upon a challenge of a lifetime. He wanted to walk around the world, touching all seven continents, in a loop starting from his home in Glasgow. Three years after waving goodbye to his class, he was within touching distance. He was walking and wild camping through nearby Glencoe in the Scottish Highlands. He would be back in his hometown in a matter of days. Sadly, it was the worst year on record for midges, a tiny fly with an intensely itchy bite. With only 90 miles to go out of 15,000, his arms and legs weeping with blood from his fingernails, he gave up. He couldn't handle the midges. It's been estimated the midges cost the Scottish economy more than £250 million every year in lost tourism and this story will do little to help.

I wasn't a sadist for walking in the Scottish Highlands naked at dusk. Yes, I wanted to get bitten. But I wanted to experience first-hand how Scotland's least popular animal and its mosquito close cousin could help doctors like me and patients like Bill.

And so, naked on that island dusk evening, with a crazed smile, I waited. Yet, nothing. No pain. Deflated, I walked back into Red Cottage and then I understood. One hundred red, circular, intensely itching bubbles on my skin. More whisky, a peat-coloured cold bath and then I thought how did they do this? Painless injections?

Needles are almost synonymous with medicine. Moments after birth, vitamin K is injected into your thigh. Then vaccinations, painkilling injections, operations as an adult, epidurals when giving birth and blood tests into older age. Life is filled with needles even for the healthy. For the ill like Bill, every hospital visit would involve countless sizes, types and places for steel darts to be inserted. And if you develop diabetes, like the 400 million or 9 per cent of adults worldwide, needles form a massive part of your life.

At medical school, most practical procedures we learn involve needles – taking blood, giving blood, antibiotics, spinal taps, lines into arteries, veins, painkilling injections, nerve blocks, biopsies.

Needles are also a common reason why people don't seek medical help. The most common fear, needle phobias can prevent vaccinations and blood tests to find diseases like cancer early. Just as the danger of falling comes from the floor not the height, it is the pain of putting the needle in, not the needle itself, which people fear. So, let's learn from my 100 bites and find out how the deadliest animal in the world can take the prick out of injections.

The deadliest creature in the world weighs the same as a small raindrop. It lives for just fifty days and has been around for 210 million years. Risking igniting a gender war, girls are the problem. It is only the female that bites, transmitting the malaria parasite after it passes through the female mosquitoes during its life cycle. After biting humans, it spits out anticoagulants including heparin to keep the blood flowing, containing malaria that kills 1 million people per year, many children. Other diseases from Zika to dengue are also transmitted this way. Girl power.

Like the Scottish midge, the secret to mosquitoes' success is that the bite is initially painless. The subsequent itch is caused by the anticoagulant in its spit, but by then it is all over. Unlike even the most skilled phlebotomist, you don't even feel a small scratch.

The mosquito had a 210-million-year head start compared with medical needle development. They were feeding from the T. rex while humans were still fish, swimming in the ocean. The hollow needle is a surprisingly modern invention. Although thin quills attached to animal bladders were described in the fifth century BC, they were mainly used for flushing out wounds rather than injections. An eleventh-century Egyptian ophthalmologist did use a hollow needle tool to remove cataracts rather than put drugs into the body. British architect Sir Christopher Wren first gave drugs using a hollow goose quill in the seventeenth century. Injecting opium and alcohol as part of anaesthesia experiments, his subjects would become 'sleepy, very drunk and then very dead'.*

Without true hollow needles, Edward Jenner's emerging science of vaccination needed to use skin cuts to inoculate children with cowpox to prevent smallpox. Anaesthesia could not advance until hollow needles were possible and pain relief or antibiotics could be reliably injected into our blood.

Conveniently for my Highland midge-biting trip, it was a Scottish surgeon, later the president of the Royal College of Physicians of Edinburgh and a member of the Royal Society, who invented the modern needle. Dr Alexander Wood called his invention the 'subcutaneous' rather than 'hypodermic' needle, a term later coined by English doctor Charles Hunter and hated by Wood. His invention was the first fine, hollow bore needle attached to an all-glass syringe. The plunger allowed careful measurement of an injection drug into the tissues or blood stream.

Wood's first patient was an eighty-year-old woman suffering from nerve pain. Hoping to relieve her pain, he injected twenty drops of vinous solution of morphia (morphine dissolved in sherry wine) into her shoulder. She went into a deep sleep but later recovered.

---

* Quoted in an article from the BBC titled 'The invention that made mass vaccinations possible' by Magnus Bennett, 9 March 2021.

The modern-day hypodermic needle has changed remarkably little from the original design. But Wood was a copycat; he stole the design from another high-flyer – the bee.

Surgeons are still learning from creatures that buzz and sting. The parasitic wasp predated human surrogate pregnancy by many millions of years. It uses an ultra-thin flexible hollow needle to insert its eggs into other insects such as beetles. This sting is like the Swiss Army knife of the insect world, also able to paralyse victims and even drill through wood.

The organ is too thin to use muscles to achieve this or move its eggs. Instead it uses friction created by a series of tiny blades that join together with a tongue-and-groove mechanism to inject eggs.

A prototype, developed by researchers in the Netherlands, has replicated this technology. It can use friction forces created by tiny moving parts to pull items up into the device. This could be used in human keyhole surgery, accessing previously hard-to-reach areas where current suction methods fail due to the small tube sizes or blockages from blood clots. This may vastly reduce the trauma from surgery and improve the recovery time of patients. Perhaps there isn't always a sting in the tail.

Remembering Johnny Cash's struggles with diabetes, on his cover of the Nine Inch Nails' song 'Hurt', he sings: 'The needle tears a hole.'

And it does. For Cash and the 400 million people with diabetes needing to prick their finger more than six times a day and inject insulin. It is this skin tearing that fires delicate pain sensors in response to skin damage by Wood's needle and then causes pain. Yet, naked in the Scottish Highlands, the only pain I felt as the midges attacked was in my foot, stepping on a thistle on the ground. A hundred bites, blood being sucked out by another life form, yet no pain. In the bath afterwards, I scratched until my skin bled but at the moment of injection I felt nothing. The needle didn't tear a hole.

A Japanese team of scientists, using super high-definition cameras and laser-guided pressure models, think they know why. The mosquito's mouth is made from several inter-twined parts. The outer tube-like straw houses two jagged saw-like jaws either side of a central needle. Although this sounds terrifying, it is using these different parts together, in sequence, that is the key to painless needles.

As the mosquito bites, it first advances the outer tube, then the jagged teeth and only then the inner needle. This sequence is repeated hundreds of times, micron by micron, until the whole structure is beneath the skin. By distributing the force in this way, spread over different parts of the skin, the force needed to penetrate is greatly reduced.

At the same time, the whole mouth vibrates at 30–40Hz in time with each advance. This gentle buzzing does two remarkable things. First, it reduces further the force needed to penetrate the skin. Second, its vibration activates skin sensors, which are different from pain sensors. Similar to TENS machines, it uses the same vibration frequency used with chronic and labour pain, which tricks the spinal cord into processing only the vibration rather than the pain.

The Japanese team has now replicated many of these features in a silicon microneedle with a three-dimensional sharp tip and harpoon-like jagged edges. Tests suggest vibrating this needle at the same frequency as the mosquito may allow true pain-free injections to be possible soon. It would help diabetics, needle phobics, children and patients like Bill, who had hoped that the tests done on his last hospital visit would be the last after being given his life back. But for Bill, life has a sting in the tail. As for me, the burn of the bites on my body receded with whisky and with time.

9

SEEING IN THE DARK

Ten years after developing cancer, Bill was cured thanks to ground-breaking CART-T treatment. A decade after that, Bill joined millions of others struck down by another deadly problem beginning with C – COVID. As the pandemic raged in Bill's hometown, it raged in villages and towns, cities and metropolises the world over. It also turned my life upside down. We needed a superhero to help. Not a nurse or a doctor, but Batman.

I used to love house parties. In my student days, we would open a big bag of crisps, serve bad wine and even worse cocktails. When middle age arrived, crisps morphed into canapes and bad wine into better craft beer. Mixing random discarded spirits became espresso martinis with a coffee bean on top.

In 2020, I was at the worst house party in history – working in ICU during the pandemic. We had more guests than we could handle, the house was too small, the packet of crisps empty, we had run out of wine and people just wouldn't go home. When all we wanted to do was sleep, we had to stay up and dance. The morning after never came, the mess got messier and neighbours complained about the noise. For two years, my phone autocorrected every capital 'W' to 'Will be home late again sorry x'.

One of the uninvited guests to this dreadful party was poor Bill. He had survived cancer, survived an experimental treatment. He had got through hyperinflammation and then toured the country with his new-found life. Yet COVID-19 would steal the end of his story as it would countless others'.

However, hope remained. Winter always turns to spring, the daffodils always come. We had technology that could look inside patients' bodies, helping to find complications of COVID. Volunteer teams self-assembled to turn patients on to their fronts when we discovered this improved oxygen levels. And the ultimate trip switch to sever the power to this party came when ninety-year-old Margaret Keenan from Coventry was given the world's first COVID-19 vaccination.

While the world was busy blaming animals for this pandemic, it was a non-human superhero that helped make this possible. Batman without the man. Let's discover how this blood-sucking, phobia-inducing creature helped cure COVID-19.

Deep in that Welsh cave where we first started our journey, high above the 20,000-year-old reindeer drawing, was a small plum-shaped creature. Still, silent, oily black. Getting permission to enter the cave had been tricky. The ecologist had insisted on a negative COVID-19 test, face masks and proof of my vaccination status.

'Don't worry,' I emailed jovially. 'I work in the ICU with COVID patients so the cave is less risky than going into work!'

'No,' came the reply. 'We aren't worried about you getting COVID. We don't want the rare bats to catch it.'

Bats could help us care for patients with COVID-19 during waves one, two and still counting, three. But it all started with a crazy Italian priest.

In 1794, self-taught scientist and Catholic priest Lazzaro Spallanzani swept a net through the air while clinging to the bell tower of a cathedral in Pavia. This wasn't the craziest thing he had done. Years before, he proved sperm was needed for frog reproduction by putting tight pants on male frogs. His latest obsession began after blowing out a candle one night – the church owl flew straight into a wall while the bats kept flying safely. Spallanzani then hung a maze of string with bells attached, proving bats could fly in the dark without making the bells ring. Covering the bats' eyes then blocking their ears with grease, he discovered it was sound not light that was the key. Yet he couldn't explain why people shouting or singing in the church didn't disturb this ability.

We now know that echolocation uses high-frequency sound emitted by bats to track objects based on the time delays for them to return. Singing or shouting at normal lower frequencies below 20kHz would make no difference, as Spallanzani had found.

How could this bat-brained idea now help look inside the bodies of patients with COVID-19? The sinking of the *Titanic* in 1912 helped. A sonar machine designed to detect icebergs in response to the tragedy used low-frequency sound waves based on bat echolocation. Further adaptations allowed Austrian Dr Karl Theodore Dussik to use ultrasound to diagnose tumours of the brain in 1942. He turned vibrations made by sound waves into image slices through the body. Finally, it was improvements in metal flaw detectors used in Scottish shipyards that made ultrasound a key tool for doctors. Bats today help you charge your toothbrush or phone without plugging it in. They help you park your car and stop it from getting stolen. We look at the unborn faces of our children thanks to bats and the *Titanic*. Ultrasound now helps me look inside patients' bodies for blood clots and infections like those caused by COVID-19. And if we find clots, bats can even help dissolve them.

What came first, Dracula or bats? Although Vlad Dracul, to give him his full name, was more than 450 years old, bats beat him wings down by 50 million years. Bram Stoker's 1897 story did solidify the links between these two creatures of the night; however, blood-drinking vampires originated in the early 1500s around Europe. Vampire fear exploded during the Great Plague with bubonic infection often causing blood to drip from people's mouths. Darwin was the first to witness a bat drinking blood during his famous voyage of the *Beagle* in 1832. After a ten-hour horse ride to Coquimbo in Chile, what become known as a vampire bat was removed from between his horse's shoulders then Darwin sketched it. So bats are named after vampires rather than the other way around.

Bats don't really suck our blood – they lap it up instead, which is perhaps even more disturbing. After making a small incision with their razor-sharp teeth near an artery, as blood trickles out, bats lick it like a cat drinking milk. Rather than screeching in pain, you would hardly notice if you were bitten. Like a skilled surgeon, bats head straight to your blood vessels. Not because they know anatomy but by using heat-seeking sensors between the eyes. Machines based on these principles have been developed to improve taking blood from patients.

Bats also spit before swallowing. Our blood-clotting system is marvellous at stopping us bleeding to death. Bats need to prevent this process to have a decent meal. After biting, they spit saliva into the wound containing the wonderfully named substance Draculin. This protein stops our most powerful clotting factors, IX and X, from building plugs that would normally stop bleeding, ensuring an eat-as-much-as-you-like buffet for the bat. Millions of people now take oral drugs based on Draculin to thin their blood instead of using older agents like warfarin that need close monitoring.

Just after I've shown how bats can save your life, let's travel to the Achuar villages near the Morona River. The mushy-pea-green, winding, thick jungle river is home to native Yankuntich and Uncun communities, nearly 700 miles north of Lima in Peru. It is not uncommon for young children to die in these tribes from what many call witchcraft. The real cause is much worse. Twelve children as young as eight died in 2016 after a spree of vampire bats were feeding on humans after livestock numbers decreased due to deforestation. The children died not from the teaspoon of blood taken while they slept, but from the subsequent rabies that was passed between bat and human in the saliva along with Draculin.

To prevent further outbreaks, two strategies have been tried. First – kill a lot of bats. This is difficult to do and rocks a delicate ecosystem. Although preserving blood-lapping, rabies-infected bats doesn't sound ideal, they are critical for global health. Bats eat flies, moths and other insects, controlling their populations. Without this, crops would soon be destroyed. Bats also serve as pollinators and seed dispersers for many plant species essential to humanity and to the tribes in this remote region. The second strategy maintains bat populations and mirrors what much of the world is trying to achieve right now – widespread vaccination.

Yesterday, I stepped back into the past. After eighteen long, PPE-shaded, grief-layered months of the pandemic, my ICU once again has lines of patients rolled on to their fronts. COVID-19 is back for a third time unlucky. The risk factors are similar yet different. Mostly patients in this third wave are again obese, diabetic, with high blood pressure. But they have one new additional characteristic, or rather lack of it. They are unvaccinated. By choice.

Many have decided that the risks of a little-known virus, already responsible for millions of deaths in a pandemic, are lower than the risks of a purpose-built, sterile, engineered vaccine already safely used by many millions more. It is easy to get mad at work, seeing the effects of one bad decision playing out again and again. I remind myself to be mad at the liars and not at the lied to. Could blood-lapping bats help us better deploy vaccines and end COVID-19 waves before they become a regular tide?

Scientists travelled to the jungle in Peru where the children died. Rabies vaccines, like the human polio inoculation, can be given orally. Bats, like many social creatures, use grooming as a key part of relationship-building. Scientists used fluorescent dyes in the vaccines to track their spread in vampire bats through grooming. The bats would light up in the night as they spread the dye along with the vaccination as they kissed, fed and cleaned each other using their mouths. Thanks to this close contact, oral and skin applied vaccines can now protect nearly three times as many bats from rabies than non-spreadable vaccines, preventing human illness and human loss.

Exploiting close social contacts that make COVID-19 so transmissible may hold the key to stopping it. Adapting similar techniques to bat rabies in diseases like COVID-19 may reduce the deaths of millions. Topical and oral vaccines are in development. Similar strategies have been used for oral vaccination in Kenya for cholera – in five days, volunteers going door to door vaccinated around 1.2 million people. The vaccine-hesitant – including the dancing, kissing, partying, young – may benefit especially from vaccination that can be passed on. Perhaps your life really can be saved by a kiss from a prince or a princess.

Even if bats can't prevent everyone from developing COVID-19, their hanging around may help those critically ill following infection. The world changed around 5 million years ago when early hominids lifted their gaze from the ground and stood upright. The benefits of standing tall are still uncertain even though this change happened before an expansion in brain size. Some suggest climate change altered African forests, making it harder and more time-consuming to find food. Evolving to use free arms and hands to grasp and carry food in enlarging open stretches between tree canopies may have helped. The impact stand-ing had on human bodies was immense. It changed the shape of our pelvis, making childbirth tougher and riskier. It rocketed our blood pressure to get blood to our higher brain. It changed the biomechanics of our joints, making lower back pain and knee arthritis a rite of passage beyond the age of fifty. It also changed every breath we take.

For years, it remained a mystery why TB mainly affected certain parts of our lungs. Initial infection attacks the bottom lobes, while TB can remain dormant for decades in the upper lung, especially on the right side. This riddle can be solved if we consider bats that, rather than evolving to stand up, evolved to hang upside down.

When we breathe in, more breath heads to the bases of our lungs. Experiments in space show gravity stretches the bottom of the lung differently to the top. This is why TB initially affects the bottom parts of the lung, being where most particles will land.

Gravity also affects blood, reducing flow to the top of the lungs. Due to how oxygen is exchanged with haemoglobin, reduced blood flow increases the oxygen levels at the top of the lung by 50 per cent. The right lung receives blood from bent vessels, further reducing flow, resulting in even higher oxygen levels. TB thrives in oxygen-rich environments, preferring this upper-right location.

Solving this 100-year-old puzzle couldn't have been

simpler. It didn't need space travel but rather a trip to that Welsh cave. Four-legged animals such as horses have dormant TB in the parts of the lung closest to the sky. While in bats, who spend their time upside down, dormant TB is found at the top and active infection at the bottom, the exact opposite of humans, as would be expected if gravity played a factor. Understanding these lung changes according to an animal's position helped us stumble across a new way to increase oxygen levels in patients critically ill with COVID-19.

With the hospital already on its bruised knees by late autumn, Christmas would bring an unwanted gift. A colleague reminded me during wave one that there's never been a day that lasts for ever. Sadly, it was starting to feel like we were in Groundhog Day after all. We had been treating COVID-19 like a sprint race in wave one. Now it was a marathon. Soon it would become an ultra-marathon where someone keeps moving the finish line. Just as infections were again rising, the government decided to give the country a jolly good knees-up, allowing families in most areas to meet over the festive season. Groucho Marx was right: Christmas doesn't come with a Sanity Clause.

Sadly, making the wrong decision was not just for Christmas. There were many empty chairs around tables as the more deadly second wave ripped through the cold winter heart of the UK. Across the Atlantic, Bill returned to the hospital where he had his world-changing cancer treat-ment. His cancer wasn't back. This time it was COVID-19.

My overwhelming memory of Christmas 2020 was not the normal late afternoon indigestion or forgetting batteries for children's presents, but bats. Walking through the inten-sive care unit over Christmas, I couldn't see patients' faces because they were all upside down, lying on their fronts.

Understanding the patterns of TB in bats helped predict how turning patients with COVID-19 on to their fronts may help oxygen levels. The backs of their lungs were becoming scarred and bruised from life support machines forcing in air. Turning patients over allowed air to enter new, undamaged parts. It changes the way blood flows and air enters, increasing oxygen levels in many patients from deadly low to survivable. This lesson has been learnt the hard way. The technique was only described in the 1970s and was not widespread until a major study was published in 2014. That is understandable. Applying lessons learnt from bats directly to large mammals like humans is not intuitive. Yet had we asked the gamekeepers of Kenya, they could have told us decades before.

You wouldn't want to sleep next to a 700kg rhino. Lying on its back, the sheer weight of its tissues and airway shape would produce loud snoring. The sound would soon be replaced with silence. Because the rhino would be dead.

Gamekeepers in Namibia noticed rhinos were dying from the effects of sedation and long journeys between grazing habitats. They brought in helicopters to speed up the transfers but still – many dead rhinos. A simple innovation would change this. The rhinos were being transported on their sides on heavy stretchers attached by a long rope to a helicopter. Attaching this strap instead to the rhino's legs, with them then dangling upside down under the helicopter, changed the way the lungs expand and the blood flows. Rhinos stopped dying. Gamekeepers knew what doctors didn't.

We have followed Bill's journey as a cancer survivor. Back in hospital with COVID-19, his oxygen levels plummeted. Years before, Bill was too early to benefit from the steroids and immune drugs that could have treated his hyperinflammation. Ironically, these exact same drugs – steroids and the immune drug tocilizumab – were shown to save lives in COVID patients but only months after Bill had been taken ill. Doctors tried ways of increasing his oxygen levels. He was rolled into different positions like bats and rhinos. But it wasn't enough. Let's travel to the steaming hot Croatian summer to meet an animal with the wind in its hair that may just help.

10

THE WIND ON YOUR FACE

If the thermometer had been an inch longer, we would have roasted to death. Krka waterfalls, chiselled out of Croatian rock, on a throbbing hot day. The powdery ground puffs underfoot with each step on the steep climb to the sound of water. Crickets sing loudly, remaining invisible. We look for elusive shade and tissue-paper-weak breeze.

Halfway through the climb, a lone flower lady stands under a frail, bony tree. Branches cast thin shadows on yellow flowers. No one buys flowers today. The heat strengthens, a migraine of sun beating down. Yet it is so beautiful. Green-glass water in the rivers hold fish still. Swallows dip, touch and fly skywards. A band of traditional harmonic Croatian singers, a suntanned version of a Welsh choir, encourage T-shirt-sweat-soaked tourists up the final ascent. Lines of people arranged like ants climbing the hill just to get to the top. But what a top it was.

Crashing white water into a flood of blue. The heat felt cooler, everything looks better with a view. I was accidentally in love with this horribly hot, beautiful place. Then it swooped down.

I grew up in a small coal-scarred industrial town in the cleavage of the Welsh Valleys. Life had a comforting pattern – school, ride your bike, hang out in a park, Saturday night into town. If the fake IDs didn't get us into The Ives pub, there were few other places to go. The nearby phone box was our consolation.

A poster inside claimed a new premium phone directory service could answer any question. That would have to be the evening's entertainment. After the obligatory 'What is the meaning of life?' question had been asked, it was my friend's turn. Nathan had a spectacular memory for contrarian facts.

'What is the fastest animal in the world?' he asked the operator who was still humouring us.

It seemed too simple. The cheetah, surely? Presumably this was the answer given by the operator, but Nathan was having none of it.

'Nope. Wrong! Only the eleventh fastest!' he said.

'Two more tries or we get our money back!'

'No, not the lion either. That's only nineteenth! Last try!'

'HAHA! The eagle. Close, second, but WRONG AGAIN! We've got you. Return our pound please!'

A small victory in a small town but the real answer has stayed with me for twenty-five years. It was the peregrine falcon, the bird I had travelled to see on that sunburnt-hot day, sweeping down above the crashing Krka waterfall. And this falcon may help Bill, lying on his front wearing an oxygen mask that was doing little for the COVID-19 he was trying to beat.

The peregrine falcon is a North American hawk, 'per-egrine' from the Latin for 'wanderer' after its migratory patterns. It is the fastest animal in the world, with speeds during dives reaching 240mph. Although the fastest, it can't claim the record for the highest flight. This goes to the griffon vulture.

Eating a pre-packed meal with plastic cutlery at 37,000ft during a flight, the last thing you would expect to see out of the plane's window is a bird. Yet sightings at this alti-tude are common. The highest ever recorded bird struck a commercial cargo plane's windscreen at 40,000ft on 19 May 2014 over Indiana. The pilot of the 767, calmly but with a chuckle in his voice in the audio recording to the control tower, said: 'Believe it or not we just had a bird strike up here. Left windshield, we're okay. We do have guts on the windshield and the outer pane is cracked. He must have been on oxygen.'

At this altitude, extracting oxygen from the atmosphere when it's just one-fifth of that at sea level is remarkable. Simply inhaling jet streams' particulate matter, like Barry's unfortunate Hobnob incident that started my animal obses-sion, should be life-threatening. I often spend time in ICU directing a fibre-optic camera deep inside lungs, pulling out bits of food from patients after a drug overdose or broken teeth after a car accident. Yet, to answer the original question posed at the start of the book: why don't birds choke on biscuits or flies or anything else?

It is because birds have a coaxial breathing system. Rather than air just going in and out of one tube, breath in birds goes around and around. Bits of Hobnob would go in but then come out. Even if they did get lodged, the multiple areas of gas exchange in a bird's lungs allow oxygen to still be extracted.

This system of circular breathing, better than any didgeridoo player's, has other advantages. In the moments before the 1.2-metre-long vulture struck the plane, its blood oxygen levels would be only a fraction lower than yours at ground level. To achieve this, it has a form of haemoglobin like human babies that adapts to low oxygen levels in the placenta. This encourages oxygen to move across from lower pressure air into the bird's blood. Their coaxial breathing system also ensures fresh air continually washes past fresh blood ready to pick up precious oxygen. That is why a griffon vulture could quite happily inhale a Hobnob even at 40,000ft and not end up in the ICU, unlike Barry.

Although we cannot change the anatomy of human lungs to match the griffon vulture, lessons from the peregrine falcon's 240mph dive can be used to care for patients like Bill tiptoeing at the edge of life with COVID-19.

As I creak into my forties, my international sports career is long behind me. Representing your country is much easier in a game that hardly anyone else your age plays. My passion was for squash – a classic sport of the 1980s played by office workers hoping to get a promotion by letting their unfit boss beat them. Although my racket is now in the attic, I try to keep fit in other ways.

Since joining CrossFit, I've learnt a lot about optimising my breathing. Especially the day I was out-weightlifted by a 76-year-old lady with two hip replacements and cancer. At the end of that session, I adopted three different positions to regain my composure. Think back to the last time you did a hard run or training session. At the end, where did you put your hands? What did you do?

First, I laid on the floor. After being helped to my feet, I leant forwards, resting my palms on my thighs with elbows pointing outwards like chicken wings. I breathed out through pursed lips, extending my breath to the very end. Then, after a few minutes, I stood upright, with my hands splayed outwards on my hips. Nearing the top of the water-fall, I adopted these positions before the final push. Why?

The simple act of lying down radically changes the air and blood flow to my lungs, improving oxygen supply to tissues, just like the rhino dangling upside down at the end of a rope.

Splinting my chest increases the amount of air in my lungs at the end of a breath. Called the functional residual capacity, this is an oxygen store that can replenish aching muscles and even help critically ill patients live. Pressing lips together increases the pressure in my lungs at the end of a breath. This positive end exploratory pressure (or PEEP) will similarly act to improve gas exchange. Walk into any emergency department and you will see patients with asthma or chronic obstructive pulmonary disease (COPD) in these positions. In bed, they will often brace against a table and purse their lips tightly.

We have machines that can artificially induce many of these lung changes in patients who are critically ill. Continuous positive airway pressure (CPAP) machines have been used by millions during the pandemic. Research shows they can reduce the need for life support machines and may save lives. Factories in industries from vacuums to aeroplane manufacturers quickly changed their production lines in early 2020 to try to meet the increased demand.

However, the tight-fitting masks needed for both machines are uncomfortable and poorly tolerated. They cause damage to the nose and prevent eating, drinking and talking. An alternative technique called high-flow nasal oxygenation can now be used, first developed in 1985 not for humans but horses. A tight-fitting mask is clearly not an option for a long-faced 1-tonne racehorse. So, a new technique was introduced to prevent exercise-induced lung bleeding, common in elite racehorses. It was widely adopted by humans a decade later and, while it's not as good as CPAP, it may help improve oxygen levels. Pushing air rapidly up the nose, it feels like skydiving at double the normal speed, just like the peregrine falcon.

But first a confession. A year after my vegetarian enlightenment on the way to Bali, I ate bacon. Here's why.

Two people with the surname 'Singer' have ruined my Christmases. The first: Professor Mervyn Singer, a leading researcher who examined my PhD. I'd spent three years trying to explain the immunology of sepsis. I foolishly thought who better to quiz me on this topic than the world expert. Big mistake. It was like three hours of *Who Wants to Be a Millionaire?*, with no lifelines, no money for right answers and very few right answers. The major revision that followed was perfectly timed to replace the festive eggnog, TV repeats and board games missing essential pieces that made a normal family Christmas. Although scientists may not enjoy criticism, the process of science thrives on wrong answers. Changes and U-turns show that science works rather than is broken. These new festive plans ultimately made my research much, much better. Professor Mervyn Singer was right.

The second Singer hasn't ruined just one Christmas, but all my future Christmases. In his mid-seventies now, Melbourne's Professor Peter Singer has wisps of white hair but solid, strong eyebrows. His Jewish parents had emigrated from Vienna. His mum was a doctor with a special interest in teaching patients with mental health problems, and his dad, despite being a coffee lover, started a tea import business after being told 'Australians don't drink coffee'. To expand his business, he wrote magazine articles in the 1940s explaining how to properly brew coffee, and may even have started a revolution resulting in the flat white that I'm drinking right now.

I read Peter Singer's book *Practical Ethics* while studying medical law before becoming a doctor. Unlike the vague paragraphs of 'maybes' in traditional ethics books, Singer's did as promised – provided solid answers to difficult, practical, ethical dilemmas. Like an annoying summer holiday song, Singer's arguments burrow deep inside your brain. They are like mind worms – so hard to remove because they remain so logically coherent.

However, it was the paradigm-shifting *Animal Liberation*, published in 1975, that led to my thesis 'The Vegetarian Vivisectionist'. I argued that, although morally acceptable to continue animal experimentation in very limited settings, eating meat could not be justified. I had conveniently forgotten this outcome, or at least embraced moral hypocrisy, until I visited Bali fifteen years later.

Singer had had animals as pets since childhood. At university, he was given an ex-laboratory rat by someone who worked there. Naming it Ratatouille long before the Disney movie, it would crawl under his jumper and sit on his shoulder. A lunch with Canadian student Richard Keshen changed Singer's life and the lunches of millions that followed. Keshen, now a professor at Cape Breton University, opted for a salad because the spaghetti sauce contained meat. The discussion that followed meant the spaghetti sauce was the last meat Singer ate.

Although Singer's reasons for promoting vegetarianism are varied, his prime argument is to avoid suffering in animals that can feel pain.

'Pain is pain,' he tells me logically, dispassionately. 'The importance of preventing unnecessary pain and suffering does not diminish simply because the being is not a human being.'

Any reasons to the contrary put forward, he argues, are nothing more than speciesism. Racism, sexism, ageism or any other ism is an unfair view based on irrelevant characteristics. So too is the treatment of non-human animals when the reasons are based only on their species rather than their ability to suffer.

Although pain is the bedrock for why eating animals should be avoided, the list goes on. Animal meat production is the most wasteful way of making food. Even chickens, the most efficient animals, need nine calories of feed to produce just one calorie of output. That is nine times the water, land, feed and pesticides. Red meat is much worse. That is even before considering the chains of shipping, feed production and slaughterhouse mechanisms. Meat production contributes nearly 15 per cent to global climate change on top of the effects of animal waste on the physical environment, such as the dead zones where nothing lives around river washouts from industrial meat manufacturing plants.

Many entirely healthy farm animals are given antibiotics every day of their lives. That is why animal meat production contributes to over 70 per cent of all antibiotic use. Given that antibiotic resistance has been described as 'the death of modern medicine' and the 'world's greatest threat' by the World Health Organization, this alone should be enough to change our direction.

Yet despite this, our demand for animal flesh goes up and

up each year. We will need more than double the amount of meat production by 2050 if the current trend continues. Oh, and by the way, animal meat production is also the most likely route to the next pandemic. Please, let's not have COVID 2.0.

That is how Peter Singer helped to ruin my future Christmases. And for that I am very grateful. I want to interact with animals in life and not on my dinner plate simply because they taste nice. Yet I ate a bacon sandwich.

It was the end of a long day, three patients under forty had died of COVID-19 in one shift. Their children had seen their mums and dads, held their hands and said good-bye and I love you. Perhaps that bacon was a crutch to the past, my past, a world past without COVID, maybe it was just because it tasted good and I had seen enough human suffering that day to blinker me to animal suffering. But that is okay. I am no moral superhero. I have done things in life I am not proud of, and I would not tell my children. I have had days when I behaved badly. But that is okay too. We all have those days.

The key is to have fewer days like that next year com-pared with this year. Over 90 per cent of people who buy meat alternatives are not vegetarians but reducers, people who feel the weight of climate change, of ethics and of animal suffering. But they are not moral superheroes either. So they try their best. If I go to a friend's house and they have cooked steak, I'll eat it. But my default, thanks to Singer's mind worm, is to go for mushrooms not meat, animal pleasure over pain, a safer world over a tastier world.

We are close to meat alternatives being cheaper and equally as tasty as animal meat. Even the major meat manufacturers have said: 'If we could make meat without the animal, why wouldn't we?' And so, even discounting the ethical arguments, plant- or lab-grown proteins can be cheaper, better and safer.

And I hope bringing these animals to life in this book will get you to think about them not as a species or a non-human but as life living alongside us. And to think of medicine not as veterinary medicine or human medicine, but as One Medicine. Now back to the peregrine falcon.

High above the Krka falls, the solitary bird looks at tourists swimming, eating ice cream then back upwards towards the sky. Its laser vision spots a blackbird circling far below. The falcon starts its dive. In just seconds it goes from zero to 240mph. More than 15g of force, double that experienced by a fighter pilot. The air rushes around its face like it would if you put your head out of the window of a jumbo jet taking off. This rushing air opens the bird's lungs further, adding positive end expiratory pressure, adding oxygen to its tissues as it plummets to earth. But the rush of air could damage its eyes, ears and lungs. It doesn't. Why not?

In 1985, a new machine was developed – for horses. To prevent the harm from tight-fitting masks, this new high-flow nasal oxygen (HFNO) technique, which blows 60 litres of oxygen-rich air a minute up the nose, moved to humans. Just like the falcon's dive, this increases the pressure in patients' airways, improving lung mechanics, increasing PEEP and improving oxygen levels. It works. But problems emerge. Patients develop damaged corneas, crusted bleeding nostrils and extreme tinnitus. It can even cause more lung damage when the flows are too high. If only we had known how the peregrine falcon deals with the wind on its face, we could have predicted this.

As the falcon reaches the middle of its dive, a series of soft flexible tissue bridges inside its nose expand to prevent lung damage. We now know to carefully regulate flow rates delivered to patients to prevent lung damage. If you could zoom in on the falcon's eyes during that dive, like a skydiver, it uses clear protective goggles. Not plastic, but a translucent third eyelid keeping its cornea's laser vision on the prey. In hospital, we now use eye protectors and gels to prevent corneal damage. As the dive reaches its maximum speed, the falcon's ears curve around like wind shields and its mouth supersaturates the air rushing in with humidification. We now offer patients earplugs and have ultrasonic humidification in the breathing machine to prevent mouth crusting. We have learnt the hard way.

We all leave a legacy whether we mean to or not. Osamu Shimomura's fireflies and jellyfish resulted in gift shops in Japan selling fluffy octopus toys as souvenirs. In 2013, Osamu saw the white parachutes dropped from the B-29

during the bombing of Hiroshima in 1945 for a second time. By now he was an old man not a schoolchild and the parachute was in the museum at Los Alamos in New Mexico where the bomb had been developed.

Osamu's son worked at Los Alamos as a computer programmer. He had invited his dad to address a specially invited audience to talk about his experience of winning the Nobel Prize. He gave the lecture to a packed audience in the very building where the technology had been designed to kill him. Just before his speech, Osamu touched the singed material of the parachute that had carried recording equipment to track the explosion he had witnessed nearly seventy years before. He ended his speech saying that it was 'unforeseen events and circumstances, scientific study, people, and chances that led to unimagined results'.

One of those unimagined results was Bill, a solider tasked with preventing another nuclear war during the Cuban missile crisis. The long hands of history stretched out from Osamu to Bill, giving him a second chance at life thanks to glowing animals and immune therapy causing a war inside his body. Bill's US Marines regiment had the motto 'King of Battle'. But all battles come to an end, all kings pass on their crown.

COVID-19 left a legacy for millions, including healthcare workers like me. Through the tough times, the teamwork, the joy and the loss, many working in healthcare, including myself, have now lived through both the day that we were born and the day that we realised why.

On 31 January 2020, 75-year-old Bill Ludwig died of

COVID-19 in the same hospital where he had received his ground-breaking cancer treatment ten years before. His memorial service was limited by pandemic precautions, but donations were to the Center for Cellular Immunotherapies. Osamu and Bill changed the world in life. The ripples their fingers made in the sea of medicine continue even after their deaths and wash over us all.

THE SEA

'How inappropriate to call this planet Earth
when it is clearly Ocean.'

ARTHUR C. CLARKE

11

HOW KISSING A FROG CAN SAVE YOUR LIFE

Casper looked remarkably well for someone who had died ten years ago. Mid-twenties, dark, round-neck T-shirt, neatly trimmed beard, sitting in front of a simple pine shelf holding a miniature bicycle and a Marshall speaker. He wore a kind smile as his melodic Danish voice told me a startling story.

'I looked very different ten years ago,' he said.

'Not just much younger, but much deader!' I replied, hoping I hadn't misjudged the humour.

Casper was one of seven children dragged from a frozen lake after a school trip went very wrong. All had been dead for over two hours before arriving at hospital. Yet, thanks to frogs, fish, whales and lizards, Casper and his friends all lived. Could medicine really reverse death after so much time has passed?

Casper's journey through reanimation started on a cold February morning. Thirteen children and two teachers set out to break a school dragon boat record on the freezing Præstø Fjord, one hour south of Copenhagen. Many students didn't want to go, but the alternative 8km run was even less appealing. When they were 2km from the shore, a gust of Arctic wind toppled the thin, yellow boat into the frozen waters.

With no radio to summon it, help was far away. From a place of fear, five children managed to swim to shore before their muscles cramped stiff from the 2°C water. Casper's sixteen-year-old friend Katherine was found wandering, confused, around a nearby forest, hypothermic and dripping wet. Soon the small town was awash with two helicopters, twelve ambulances, the coastguard and fishing boats. Casper couldn't swim. He couldn't get to the shore.

The fishermen find two boys. The coastguard spot two girls. Three children are winched by helicopter after gripping for an hour on to floating ice. All seven children are frozen still. They have no heartbeat. The ambulance calls the hospital saying all seven children are dead.

One of the first things we were taught about resuscitation as medical students was: 'You are not dead until you are warm and dead.' It has long been known that severe hypothermia can both mimic death and protect the body from cardiac arrests.

One of the more high-profile people who might have experienced hypothermia at least once during their life is

Jesus. Lying naked in a manger during winter meant baby Jesus would have got very cold, say Australian researchers.*
The temperature on 25 December in Nazareth would have been around 7°C. Although based on secondary sources hundreds of years after the event, by reviewing paintings by the Old Masters in London's National Gallery, researchers found Jesus was naked or scantily clothed in almost all of them. Neither frankincense, gold nor myrrh could have kept the Messiah warm. Hypothermia has also helped others who, like Jesus, rose from the dead.

Anne Greene was a 22-year-old servant living in Oxford. Pregnant with her master's grandson's baby, she kept it a secret. The baby died after being born prematurely and, fearing for the consequences, she hid the dead child. On 14 December 1650, Anne Greene was hanged for murder in the Oxford Cattle Yard in front of a large crowd on a freezing cold day. Drawings show family members pulling on Anne's feet, hoping to end her misery more quickly. After being cut down, her body was taken in a coffin to the laboratory of the famous Oxford University doctor, Thomas Willis.

Hours later, the coffin was opened and Anne Greene was still breathing. Willis's team used medical techniques thought to help resuscitate patients, including pouring hot liquor down the throat, tobacco smoke enemas, draining blood and tickling Anne's throat with a feather. After twelve hours in a warm bed, Anne began speaking. Twenty-four

---

* Koh, T. & Koh, M. R., 'A chilling thought for Christmas 2004: might the newborn Christ have been hypothermic?', *The Medical Journal of Australia*, **181**, 680–681 (2004).

hours later, she was answering questions freely. The court decided to grant Anne a reprieve and she later married, had children and lived for another fifteen years.

In Chapter 12 we will meet animals that regularly survive freezing conditions, hinting at how humans could extend their lives. But for young frozen Casper to even have a chance at this life, doctors first needed to help him breathe – like a frog.

Television news channels were saturated with patients on life support machines during the COVID-19 pandemic. These devices help push oxygen-enriched air into failing lungs, in the hope that time will be a healer. In 6 million years of human evolution, it is only during the last seventy that human lungs have breathed in this new, strange way.

Take a deep breath in right now and feel your diaphragm pushing down while simultaneously the muscles between your ribs contract, pulling them upwards and outwards. Together this creates negative pressure in the layers between your elastic lungs and ribcage. This pressure is transmitted to 500 million tiny air sacs inside, drawing in air. This is the moment when air becomes breath, using negative pressure to inflate your lungs.

In my first book, *Critical*, I told the story of a 12-year-old girl called Vivi, who became the world's first intensive care patient during the 1952 Copenhagen polio epidemic. Unable to breathe for herself, a hole was cut in her neck.

Medical students then squeezed a rubber bag attached to her windpipe, keeping Vivi alive by breathing in the opposite way – squeezing air into her lungs using positive pressure.

In the years since Vivi's treatment, we have learnt what this new breathing technique does to our lungs. Although life-saving for patients with diseases including COVID-19, life support machines can become death-supplying machines if used incorrectly. Early in my medical training, I saw patients die from the side effects of this new way of breathing. Our lungs are not designed to have these forces applied. Their delicate lining breaks, fractures, swells and scars from tissue shearing caused by positive pressure. Tiny air sacs burst, letting air escape around our heart, into our skin and even inflating our faces. I have inserted countless plastic tubes to prevent the build-up of excess air from crushing the heart to death.

But Brazilian water frogs, African lizards and even my dog, Chester, know how to safely use these machines. These animals have been breathing using positive pressure for more than 400 million years. And they will all help Casper.

As soon as Casper's frozen, heartbeat-less body arrived in hospital, doctors made a key decision. They decided he was not dead until he was warm and dead. They decided all seven children filling their emergency department were not dead until they were warm and dead. It was going to be a very long day. The whole hospital embarked on a remarkable journey to warm the children's blood and bodies safely: slowly. But the first step if Casper and his friends were going to survive was to protect their lungs.

A small flexible plastic tube, the size of your middle finger, was inserted between Casper's vocal cords into his breathing pipe. This tube was connected to a life support machine that squeezed pressurised oxygen-enriched air into Casper's lungs. As it did, his chest would rise and fall as breath was moved in and out. This was the first time Casper's lungs had breathed like this in his life, using positive pressure rather than negative.

Casper's team knew about the damage life support machines could do. They had helped with research showing that the key to preventing damage was to use small, 400ml breaths, about the capacity of a beer can, for the average person. This reduced the harm from stretching lungs and helped limit the air pressure. It allowed Casper and his friends to stay on life support machines safely for many days without their lungs falling apart while their blood was slowly warmed.

What the medical team didn't realise was that they were borrowing from ancient animals and remote jungle tribes to give Casper a second chance at life.

Halfway through medical school, students have six weeks away from campus to study a topic of their choice. In my year group, some voluntarily entered Cardiff's high-security jail to shadow prison doctors. Others studied wilderness medicine in the stormy Welsh mountains. I worked at a bar late into the early mornings before class to save enough money to get me to Brazil. There I worked with HIV-positive sex workers and drug addicts who filled charity hospitals run by nuns overlooking the beaches of Copacabana. I met some extraordinary characters including one the size of a pea – the tiny Brazilian gold frog.

Our meeting took place over four hours on a bumpy bus and an even bumpier boat from Rio with global strangers. My seasick eyes opened to jungle-covered hills peering down at talcum powder beaches bordering blue lagoons filled with tropical fish. We had travelled to Ilha Grande, a beautiful island with an ugly history.

First a slave trading port and then a quarantine island in the late nineteenth century for ships carrying European immigrants, Ilha Grande later housed Brazil's most dangerous criminals as a prison called Caldeirão do Diabo or Devil's Cauldron. Comando Vermelho, one of the most powerful mafias in the country, was founded on this remote island before the prison locked its gates in 1994.

A three-hour trek along winding jungle paths, strange noises around every corner, took our newly formed group of friends to Lopes Mendes, the Blue Lagoon. Despite, or perhaps due to, having no bars, no restaurants and no sun loungers, it often wins the title of the best beach in Brazil, in a country with more than 2,000 to choose from. With a caipirinha cocktail to rehydrate me after the trek back to the hostel, medical school felt a million miles away. Well, it was more than 5,000 miles away I suppose. It was then that a tiny pea-sized frog jumped almost weightlessly on to my left foot. A wild guess, I asked the Brazilian bar worker if it was the Brazilian gold frog I had read about on the bus.

'Sim,' she said through a half-smile.

'That is why this place is called The Golden Frog Hostel.'

Though small, this frog can be very aggressive. Males sometimes fight by pulling out a competitor's organs using their tongue. Although it was no match for my hiking boots, I closely watched the area under its wide mouth expanding and contracting as it breathed.

The Brazilian gold frog, like other related amphibians, has three ways to absorb oxygen and remove carbon dioxide. When underwater, their thin skin acts like an external lung. They also have a permeable lining in their mouth where gas exchange can occur. But most breathing happens using a similar mechanism to Casper's life support machine.

Like humans, frogs first pull in air through their nostrils. This expands and fills the flexible under-mouth area resulting in the classic balloon-like bulging. This air can't be sucked down into the lungs as frogs lack a powerful diaphragm. Instead, their mouth muscles contract as their windpipe opens to force air, under positive pressure, into the lungs. That tiny Brazilian gold frog on my foot was breathing just like patients on a life support machine – just like Casper.

Frogs can teach intensive care professors a thing or two.

Unlike humans, whose lungs are adapted to only negative pressure ventilation, frogs have had millions of years to perfect their technique. Both the type of airflow and the amount of breath used in frogs match exactly what scientists have recently learnt by studying thousands of humans on life support machines.

Frogs breathe using a volume of air matching that magic human number of 400ml (in proportion to their size). Plus, the flow pattern used to drive in air matches that found in modern life support machines costing hundreds of thousands of pounds. Frog breathing techniques are even used in patients like Vivi, who survived polio, to give their lungs an extra boost when their diaphragm remains weak.

Doctors caring for Casper had carefully calculated the amount of breath their life support machines were delivering using this original proportion from frogs. Every time Casper's chest rose upwards, the bright monitors showed airflow patterns mirroring that tiny frog on my foot. It was as if Casper was kissing a frog to help save his life, using just the right amount of air.

It's not only kissing a frog that can save your life. In many serious lung conditions, even breathing 100 per cent oxygen using a life support machine may not help. During crushingly busy pandemic night shifts, patients' oxygen levels would frequently plummet below 70 per cent, lower than levels in some climbers without oxygen at the top of

Everest. It would be as if they were passengers on a terrible, turbulent flight as the aeroplane suddenly depressurised. We would have only minutes to think of new ways to keep these patients alive. Thankfully, dogs and lizards helped.

After rushing to a patient's bedside, I would press buttons and turn knobs on their life support machine, trying different methods to inflate their lungs. One novel way of breathing I would use, developed in 1987, was airway pressure release ventilation (APRV). Try it yourself. Take a deep breath in right now and then have a big, long laugh or a long cry. You will start taking rapid, small breaths in and out with each laugh or cry at the top of that first inhalation. Congratulations, you have just activated APRV mode without the months of training that it normally takes doctors. This technique can increase oxygen levels even in the sickest patients with diseases like COVID-19.

Don't feel too proud of yourself just yet, though – the bedouin spiny-tailed lizard beat you to it by around 220 million years, long before COVID-19 closed borders and minds. This exact type of breathing is used periodically by lizards to help them deal with dry and sandy conditions that would otherwise drop their oxygen levels like our patients' during night shifts.

I've promised to include my dog, Chester, in every book I write. Thankfully, dogs really can help us here too. The final machine I sometimes wheel out at night is called the high-frequency oscillator. This noisy, bulky device was developed in the 1970s to treat premature babies but can be used in critically ill adults. If you stand close to the stage at a heavy metal concert, you will understand how it works. Like a powerful speaker, it has a flexible diaphragm vibrating quickly to fire shock waves into lungs. This oscillates or jiggles air, increasing blood oxygen levels in some people, although the machine does tend to explode when used incorrectly. This doesn't help.

The device mirrors what Chester does most days without being a trained doctor and without the explosion risk. After losing yet another ball in long grass, Chester will sit looking at us longingly while panting. His pants, although mainly used for heat loss, add oxygen to his blood using the same physics principles as the oscillator. Although the initial settings I enter on the machine are difficult to remember, especially at night, Chester knows them well. He pants using the exact same frequency as I dial up for patients – 5Hz, or 300 breaths per minute.

Thankfully, Casper didn't need exploding machines or lizard breathing. He just needed his lungs to be kept safe by breathing like a frog. But the plastic pipe between his vocal cords did need to stay in place for a long time without Casper coughing. To find out how this was possible for Casper, and intensive care patients all around the world, let's travel across South America, from the home of the Brazilian gold frog to the golden poison frog in Ecuador – a frog you definitely do not want to kiss.

Fifty miles south-east of Panama City's bustling chaos is a 1 million acre tropical rainforest barely touched by deforestation. The twisting mangrove swamps and dense green canopy are home to sloths, monkeys, parrots and the reclusive Chocó tribe, living in small groups of extended families. Arriving by canoe on the Sambú River, you would first glimpse tall stilted huts with dense thatched roofs. The Chocó, first contacted by Spanish explorers in 1511, wear little more than black paint made from seeds of jagua fruit from ankle to mouth. Although they eat plentiful plantains, bananas, coconuts, mangos, guava and cocoa, valuable protein sources are scarce. Most come from dangerous animals including tapirs and crocodiles. Yet the most dangerous animal of all is also their route to survival – the golden poison frog.

The 5cm long, brightly coloured, golden metallic green frog secretes a powerful toxin from its skin. Each frog could kill twenty humans or an elephant. One gram of the toxin could kill 15,000 people. This batrachotoxin attacks sodium channels in nerve cells, causing complete muscle paralysis. The chemical was first analysed in 1971 by explorers who skinned hundreds of frogs caught with the tribe's help. Although the visitors used gloves, goggles and face masks, their expedition dog died after scavenging on poison contaminated rubbish.

Even before this chemical analysis, the Chocó had known of the toxin's powers for generations. Hunting parties would use poison-tipped blow darts, made by gently rubbing against a frog's back while held between leaves and sticks. The darts, with spiral grooves to hold the toxin, are fired from blowpipes made from two shafts of palm wood glued together with tree resin. Safely hunting even massive crocodiles from a distance is made possible thanks to a single blow dart paralysing all the animal's muscles instantly.

This frog poison has played a key part in developing muscle relaxants, heart stimulants and anaesthetics used in modern healthcare. The related compound, curare, was shown in the nineteenth century to treat tetanus spasms. In 1942, Pascual Scannone, a Venezuelan anaesthesiologist working in New York, first used a muscle relaxant like that from the poison frog to pass a flexible plastic tube through the vocal cords of a patient needing an operation.

The march of scientific progress led to related drugs being injected through Casper's frozen veins. Tubes were then safely put into his lungs and stayed there for days. His floppy muscles, paralysed like the crocodiles caught by poison frog darts, allowed life support machines to use just the right amount of breath, thanks to the kiss of another frog.

Decades later, the same muscle paralysis drugs had nearly run out during another night shift at the hospital where I worked. The whole intensive care unit was flooded with COVID-19 patients lying face down, having just the right amount of breath thanks to frogs, sometimes breathing like lizards or dogs. But there were too many patients. Too few staff. I didn't know if sunrise would come for them all. But we all pulled together. Solidarity was contagious during the early lockdowns. But now news channels flicker in staff rest areas with the fractures of division rather than the melting of togetherness. The daily stress in hospitals and communities was like a sorting hat for bastards – people you thought were friends became empty, distant or unreliable, yet others filled your boots with hope and thanks and support. Despite the amazing animals that supported our patients' fight for survival, at these dark moments it was humanity that was amazing. I often think even when individual humans are terrible, humanity remains astonishing.

12

As cold as ice

Lying in the emergency department, frozen and dead, Casper's body was inanimate. Despite tubes into his lungs attached to a life support machine, his oxygen remained low, his temperature even lower. Casper's muscles were wood-stiff from the cold, especially after muscle paralysing drugs had been given. Doctors had agreed the seven frozen children would not be declared dead until they were warm and dead. But achieving this seemed unimaginable; Lake water had filled their lungs, making survival using life support machines alone impossible.

That tragic day in Copenhagen, doctors needed to look to the deep past to improve the prospects for Casper's future – 300 million years into the past. This was when ancestors of modern fish and reptiles emerged from swamps and underwater. They had started breathing air, not liquid. Now Casper would need to hold his breath for days. Oxygen needed to be added directly to his blood, without using lungs, just as fish had done millions of years before. The icefish knows how this could be done.

Stories of a fish with icy white blood were first told when Captain Cook returned from his second voyage in 1775. Sailors in ale houses told tales of whalers catching fish so transparent that their brains could be seen through their skulls and through their scales. Unlike many fishing stories, these tales came true when one of the most remote islands on Earth was discovered.

A snow-covered rock, tiny Bouvet Island is a speck in the vast South Atlantic, 3,000 miles east of South America. After being claimed by Norway in 1927, Norwegian biologist Ditlef Rustad stayed on the island and caught a fish like no other. Large eyes, long protruding jaw full of teeth. Utterly pale, transparent, like a ghost. Rustad called it a 'white crocodile fish'. When cut open, its tissues were filled with 'blod farvelöst', he wrote in his notebook – colourless blood. It took another twenty-six years for scientists to understand how this fish could live without red blood.

The icefish has very thin blood, just 1 per cent of its volume is made from cells. Around 45 per cent of human blood is a mixture of immune white cells and oxygen carrying red blood cells. Even the 1 per cent of cells in the icefish don't carry oxygen. It is as if these strange fish have ice water in their veins.

Living in the deep ocean, at the bottom of the Antarctic sea shelf, the first mystery to solve is why icefish don't just freeze to death. At 100 metres deep, these 2ft-long prehistoric creatures are surrounded by high pressure and super-cooled water at a temperature between 2 to -2°C. We now know the blood in their veins contains anti-freeze proteins, preventing ice crystals from forming and damaging their organs. This alone could have huge advantages for the care of patients needing organ transplantation. But it doesn't explain how the icefish uses oxygen without the red blood needed to carry the gas of life.

Having different coloured blood is not unique. Insects and crustaceans use hemocyanin, a bluish copper-based pigment, to carry oxygen. Some worms use the purplish hemerythrin, some the green chlorocruorin. The colour differences represent different elements used, wrapped up in protein blankets, to carry oxygen. We often forget how utterly strange it is incorporating metal inside blood cells. The physicist Carl Sagan puts this beautifully, saying: 'The nitrogen in our DNA, the calcium in our teeth, the iron in our blood, the carbon in our apple pies were made in the interiors of collapsing stars. We are made of star stuff.'*

This star stuff can be dangerous. Haemoglobin, our oxygen-carrying compound that uses iron, is a small and reactive substance when exposed. It is so toxic that our liver makes a protein designed to neutralise any that escapes from broken cells. Haemoglobin can mute chemical messengers including nitric oxide, reduce blood flow to our organs and even block kidneys. Therefore it is normally packed away safely inside red blood cells.

Living without toxic star stuff molecules has advantages.

---

* Sagan, C., *The Cosmic Connection: An Extraterrestrial Perspective*, pp. 189, 190, Anchor Press/Doubleday, Garden City, New York, 1973.

But among 50,000 vertebrates, the icefish is unique in lacking haemoglobin and red blood cells. How can it survive? And why does understanding this strange creature help patients? Patients like Casper and Chris Lemons, a deep-sea diver, stranded at the bottom of the North Sea with no light, no heat and no oxygen?

In the blackened North Sea, 130 miles from land, extraordinary people are doing extraordinary things right now. They are grounded astronauts, exploring the depths of our own Earth. Chris Lemons was one of those people – a deep-sea saturation diver, spending his life repairing pipes most of us never knew existed.

Chris didn't plan on becoming a professional aquanaut. A chance summer job in his twenties on a dive boat led to him working on the largest commercial underwater pipelines around the world. Descending to the seabed radically changes human bodies. The incredible pressures force gasses to dissolve into the blood. Like a bottle of Champagne, quickly releasing that pressure would cause an explosion of bubbles. Unlike the fizz in the glass flute, these bubbles are not good. They could block arteries and veins, risking death. So instead, saturation divers like Chris remain under high pressure for twenty-eight days straight. They live in cramped conditions alongside other crew mates in a support ship's decompression chamber between every dive.

The job planned for 18 September 2012 should have been

just another day at the underwater office for Chris and his two colleagues. But soon after reaching the bottom of the freezing North Sea, everything changed.

One hundred metres above Chris, the surface sea became rough. Waves crashed on to the deck of the support ship that supplied warmth, light and oxygen to the divers down below. Then the positioning system that kept the ship in line with the divers failed. Red alarm lights flashed, sirens sounded, panicked faces were all around. The vessel moved further and further out of position, stretching the twisted umbilical cord linking the divers to the ship via a diving bell. Chris's colleague scrambled underwater towards the diving bell's safety just in time. But Chris's lifeline was caught around an underwater pipe. He was in trouble. The line became tighter and tighter, before first the lights went out, then his dive suit heating failed and then, with a loud bang, the lifeline snapped. Chris landed on his back, 100 metres deep in the black 2°C water, with no light, no heat and just nine minutes of emergency oxygen from tanks on his back.

The ship above had drifted half a kilometre away from the divers. The crew watched Chris's curled up body on video screens using underwater cameras. He looked like a lonely little boy. They battled the sea to rescue Chris but couldn't get there in time. On the video screens, his body twitched and water filled his helmet. Then the twitching stopped.

Thirty-seven minutes after the oxygen had run out, a diver finally reached Chris's lifeless body. It was carried to the diving bell's airlock. Resuscitation seemed cruel, but his colleague who had watched helplessly from the diving bell, blew two rescue breaths into Chris's cold, blue mouth.

Are there mysteries from the deep that could have helped Chris survive? How can some animals hold their breath for long periods? And could the icefish hold the key to life for people in a similar situation to Chris?

During a family holiday to France, we had a brush with drowning when our kayak overturned. It was a scorching day on the laid-back Dordogne river. After a stop for lunch, our two children got back on to the boat, nearly leaving the life jackets behind. Minutes later, the wide meandering river transformed into a swirling rip around a fallen tree. Sucked into the swirl, our boat flipped, sending Mimi, my youngest daughter, down the river. My wife just managed to grab the back of her life jacket and followed her down the river.

Opening my eyes after surfacing, my eldest daughter, Evie, was nowhere. Clinging on to a branch from the fallen tree, I scanned the river and bank – nothing. All that remained was our overturned kayak. Using strength I do not have, I flipped over the boat to reveal my daughter. She had a completely dry face with her hat and sunglasses still in place!

Had Evie not been harboured by the kayak's air pocket,

my daughter would have had around two minutes of life left by holding her breath. Although poorly designed for breath-holding, humans can extend this time, as the Croatian free-diver Budimir Šobat demonstrated. In 2021, he held his breath for twenty-four minutes and thirty-seven seconds, beating the previous world record by thirty-four seconds. Part of his secret was to act like a turtle.

When sleeping, turtles can stay underwater for hours. This is helped by a thin membrane in their rectum allowing turtles to breathe underwater through their arse. During hibernation in cold water, they move very little, allowing them to hold their breath for up to seven hours. When caught in nets, however, they quickly use their oxygen stores and will drown in just minutes. Free-divers similarly reduce their oxygen consumption. They meditate, slow their heart rate, relax their muscles and act much like Chris Lemons lying unconscious on the ocean floor after his oxygen supply ran out. The extreme cold that inflicted Casper and Chris automatically slows metabolic pathways, reducing oxygen consumption without the need for meditation.

Free-divers copy another aquatic animal to prolong their breath-hold even longer. If you hold your breath and plunge your face into cold water, your body triggers a primordial diving response. This primitive reflex handed on from our fish ancestors slows your heart rate and constricts blood vessels, further preserving oxygen stores. I've used this evolutionary hack on patients with an abnormally fast heart rate. Plunging their face into a bucket of ice water in the emergency department can quickly cure a life-threatening condition.

Studying the seal's response to diving, researchers showed this diving reflex also affects the spleen. You probably don't think much about this 150g organ, found on your left side behind your kidney. It contains one quarter of a litre of blood in humans or up to half the blood volume in racehorses. Seals use their spleen as a perfect back-up store of oxygen-rich blood when holding their breath for long periods. The diving response constricts the spleen, pouring extra blood into their system during a dive. Humans in free-diving communities, like the remote Filipino Bajau tribe, have much bigger spleens, helping them stay under-water for more than thirteen minutes at depths of 60 metres. Unlike humans, where repeated breath-holding, such as in conditions like sleep apnoea, leads to heart problems, seals use gases including nitric oxide and carbon monoxide to prevent high pressures developing in the blood vessels of their lungs. Step into my intensive care unit and you will see these same techniques and gases being used in patients with lung failure due to conditions from COVID-19 to sepsis.

Lying on the ocean floor, Chris Lemons was battling the same challenges as the icefish – low oxygen in his blood, high pressures and the blistering cold. The key to his survival also lay with these threats.

In your blood, 98 per cent of the oxygen is linked to haemoglobin within red blood cells. Just a tiny 2 per cent is dissolved in the watery plasma. The icefish could make haemoglobin but doesn't bother. It relies entirely on dissolved oxygen with a few tricks to make it enough to live on.

Any good bar worker knows beer is best when cold. Temperature is a key factor influencing the solubility of gas in liquids. The colder the beer, the more carbon dioxide can dissolve, giving beer that satisfying fizz. However, future space tourists on Elon Musk's rockets will be disappointed even if their beer is cold. Pressure is another element changing gas solubility – the low pressure of space travel would make even cold beer very flat.

The icefish survives thanks to the high solubility of oxygen in their watery blood, made possible by the high pressure at 100 metres deep and the freezing cold water. Although possessing still just 10 per cent of the oxygen found in red blood, they compensate in other ways. Icefish have large hearts, dense blood vessel networks and a high blood volume. This allows high flows of their thin blood with plenty of time and space for organs to extract dissolved oxygen. Icefish also use nitric oxide in their lungs, the same drug we use in critically ill patients with COVID-19, to help maximise oxygen extraction from each breath. Lying motionless for long periods on the ocean floor, filter feeding small prey, also helps in minimising their oxygen need.

In other words, the icefish is just like Chris's lifeless body – lying still at the bottom of the sea, freezing cold, under pressure. The dissolved oxygen in his blood remained high thanks to these conditions. And Chris's years of working as a saturation diver may have dramatically changed his body. Compared to the average land dweller, he had a larger volume of blood, floppier blood vessels with more nitric oxide and a larger heart. Sometimes it is more important to know what sort of person has a disease than what sort of disease they have.

Chris spent forty minutes without breathing. This should have been impossible to survive. But Chris wasn't like a normal human. He was half icefish. Maybe, just maybe, that was enough to revive his human side. Alive.

Casper's second chance at life came not from being isolated and alone, but from an emergency department filled with a team of lifesavers. Still freezing cold, doctors inserted pipes into Casper's arteries and veins. Dark, red, cold blood was pulled out from his body and pushed into a heart-lung machine where oxygen was artificially added and carbon dioxide removed. The machine gradually warmed Casper's blood, slowly, a fraction of a degree by a fraction of a degree.

Despite the added oxygen, Casper's cold blood couldn't deliver enough to his tissues. Lactic acid built up as his organs struggled to stay alive. But turning up his temperature any faster would risk a reperfusion injury, where toxins flood the body after blood flow is restored. Swamping struggling organs with oxygen-rich blood after they had been shut down for so long can make things much worse. But perhaps the carp and even the mole could help him.

Eastern moles, native to North America, have eyes

covered in skin as they spend so much time in the blackened underground. Deep underground, oxygen levels dip to 14 per cent compared with 21 per cent at the surface. Like when you breathe in and out of a paper bag to try to cure hiccups, carbon dioxide also ramps up from 1 per cent to over 6 per cent. To survive, moles have a haemoglobin that blocks a chemical called 2,3 DPG. This makes more room for carbon dioxide to bind and allows oxygen to travel more efficiently. Changes in 2,3 DPG explain why human blood transfusions struggle to carry normal amounts of oxygen, especially during treatment like that used on Casper. Patients with anaemia may benefit from drugs that increase levels of 2,3 DPG and new trials using this therapeutic target for conditions including sickle cell disease have just started.

The crucian carp, living deep in the cold seas off the Arctic Circle, shows similar changes in its haemoglobin to better bind oxygen. But it also prevents reperfusion injury after long winter hibernations by having the largest stores of energy-rich glycogen found in any vertebrate species. Its tissues can produce glucose energy without oxygen while avoiding the build-up of lactic acid that Casper was now battling. These findings have helped to explain several rare human diseases affecting metabolism where lactate levels become dangerously high during normal life. Instead, carp use a metabolic pathway that produces ethanol as a waste product – the original microbrewery. Their blood alcohol level is around about 0.05–0.1 per cent, equivalent to drinking two pints of beer.

Three weeks after Chris Lemons ran out of oxygen for forty minutes while repairing pipes on the deep ocean floor, something remarkable happened – he went back to finish the job. Those two rescue breaths pushed into his blue mouth by a colleague worked. Chris started to breathe, his eyes opened, he lived. Back on the ship, the only medical treatment Chris needed was a tea cosy on his head to keep him warm. Hours later, while the ship's medic took his pulse, Chris leant forwards and said: 'You do know it's okay, don't you? It's just like drifting off to sleep. I was sad for a bit. I was cold and got a bit numb but then it was just like falling asleep.

'It's not that bad.'

Chris was talking about dying. Apparently, it's not so bad.

His story is a remarkable feat of survival, made possible thanks to the cold, the pressure and the adaptations to Chris's body from a career of deep-sea diving. The icefish helped show us that survival even in these extremes is possible. But it isn't just deep-sea divers that could benefit from the 20-million-year-old lessons from the icefish. Its paper-like bones, so thin you can see its brain through its skull, may help millions of humans with broken hips from osteoporosis. Its white blood provides new ideas for dealing with extreme loss of blood and anaemia. And understanding how it lives in the freezing cold without actually freezing stiff can help prevent ice crystals forming in human organs waiting for a transplant.

As for Casper, his gradual rewarming using the heart-lung machine started to work. His oxygen levels crept upwards; his lactic acid started going down. The extreme 2°C cold water had slowed his metabolism just enough to protect his organs. His body temperature was recorded at a chillingly low 17°C. Both he and Chris had survived this far thanks to the very threats that could have extinguished their lives. Chris, under extreme pressure and deep cold, had just enough oxygen in his lifeless body to stop death. Casper, still on life support machines, hadn't died because he was cold and dead.

Now he was warmer and becoming more alive every minute. Six hours after the accident, at 26°C, his heart started beating. The doctors could not believe it. The waiting room filled with parents erupted. Oily tears filling the creases under their eyes. But then his heart went crazy. However, a 30-tonne whale could help fix it.

13

A HEART THE SIZE OF A PIANO

Casper's blood had reached the temperature of a cool swimming pool – just high enough for his heart to start beating, but too cold for it not to stop again. A few regular beats on the monitor in the ICU gave way to a shaky line, trembling like his parents in the waiting room. Casper's entire heart was fibrillating, twitching in a chaotic manner, useless for pumping blood. If the storm couldn't be calmed, Casper would die. Again.

Atrial fibrillation, where the top of your heart shakes, is common. The president of the United States, Joe Biden, had a shaking heart at one point. So did Elton John, Tony Blair and even 007 (Roger Moore). But when the whole heart jitters, normal life is not possible. Without the military co-ordination of heart muscles squeezing at the right times, in the right places, blood cannot get to your brain or your organs.

With Casper's heart dancing in his chest, doctors needed to fix it quickly. And they could with the help of a 30-tonne whale and its massive 180kg heart.

Frits Meijler sits back in a chair and relaxes. The smooth oil painting of him hanging in Utrecht's University Medical Center hides the adventure that ran through the veins of this pioneering heart doctor. Although a human cardiologist, Meijler had long been fascinated with the hearts of larger mammals. 'I did horses and elephants, but I needed the ultimate one – a whale.'

This obsession with whales' hearts was passed down by contemporaries including Dr Paul White, President Eisenhower's physician. White dreamt for forty years of capturing an electrical recording of a whale's heart. He came blisteringly close, only to nearly die in the process.

Medicine sometimes needs to search for answers outside of minty white laboratories, in faraway, dangerous places. National Geographic magazine described White's 1956 expedition to Mexico's Scammon's Lagoon, a remote place visited only by the occasional turtle hunter. With the sun flaming across the Mexican sand dunes, White attached an electrical wire to a huge 40ft mother whale near her calf. It didn't go well.

'The whale charged into the keel, sheared off the rudder, bent the propeller, and left the fragile craft with a gaping hole smashed in the bottom,' he told the magazine, pictured with the shattered vessel. The whale had taken off with the delicate ECG recording equipment in tow.

Thirty years later, Frits Meijler returned to Scammon's Lagoon, before calving time but during mating season. Joining the expedition was His Royal Highness Prince Bernhard of the Netherlands. Bernhard later founded the World Wildlife Fund, becoming an avid defender of the whale. He told reporters that a killer whale had once kissed him on the cheek and it felt like silk.

Meijler thought that mating season would be an ideal time to do an ECG recording as there are so many whales in close proximity. In retrospect, this probably wasn't his greatest idea as whales normally have threesomes. When mating, two males work together, one holding the other upright to aid the insertion of its Pink Floyd into the female.* Perhaps unsurprisingly, the ECG recording was unsuccessful because suckers on the end of the harpoons became detached during sex.

It wasn't until 1991 that an accurate whale's ECG was finally recorded. Tiny electrical signals from a massive 10-metre, 30-tonne humpback whale's heart were captured using 10cm-wide suckers on long poles attached to its skin. Although this obsession with piano-sized hearts seems strange, Frits Meijler explains that 'in setting forth with such an aim, we were really searching for the mysteries of the human heart'. And this voyage helped revolutionise the field of cardiac electrophysiology, understanding how electricity affects humans.

Accompanying Frits on his expedition was another

---

* If there is one piece of knowledge you take away from this book, let it be that a whale's penis is called a Pink Floyd (no link to the band).

doctor, Hein Wellens, who I spoke with shortly before his death in June 2020. Wellens, called the father of electrophysiology, pioneered many of the treatments we now use when hearts develop arrhythmias. It is thanks to Wellens and Meijler and the whale that patients, including Joe Biden and 007, can live on when their hearts are out of sync. It was thanks to this unlikely trio that Casper's heart could be saved. Because when the whale's heart tracing was analysed, it shattered theories on how hearts keep time.

A whale's heart is twice as heavy as an average human being, with the same volume as a grand piano. Contrast this to the smallest mammal heart, that of a shrew, the size and weight of a human teardrop. While the whale's heart plods along at 10–30 beats per minute, the shrew sprints at more than 800. Until the whale's ECG was analysed, it was a mystery how these two remarkable feats of engineering use the same molecular structures and biochemical pathways. It is like using the same electrical wires to power a wristwatch and a football stadium. Understanding how this is achieved was a key piece of the puzzle needed to develop treatments for when things go wrong.

The use of electricity to re-spark life predated Mary Shelley's 1818 book *Frankenstein*. Thirty years earlier, the first description of a successful resuscitation using electric shocks was reported by the English surgeon Charles Kite. In 1788, three-year-old Sophie Greenhill fell from a window on to a paved London street. Surprisingly, the neighbour who found her apparently dead decided to apply electricity to various parts of her body. Using static electricity stored in a specialised jar, he passed a current through her arms and legs. When put 'through her chest', the neighbour felt 'a small pulse, and within a few minutes the child began to breathe with great difficulty'. Sophie was restored to perfect health and spirits in about a week.

We now know how electricity can treat the abnormal heart rhythms that can cause apparent death through cardiac arrests. We have machines that deliver set amounts of electricity, in the right patterns, at just the right times to reset chaotic electrical signals. But despite using these modern machines, Casper's heart continued to shake erratically, as do millions of hearts around the world with common arrhythmias like atrial fibrillation. To treat these, doctors instead need to use electricity as more than just a reset switch. They needed to understand the complex meat-based circuitry of the heart and where to add or remove signals. They needed to understand the ECG from the heart of the 30-tonne whale recorded by Frits Meijler.

Before considering the whale's unusual ECG, the physical structure of its heart is also pretty amazing. By 2019, underwater research technology had advanced significantly since the tangle of wires used by Meijler and White. A Californian team was able to attach a wireless tag to a free-diving blue whale. During descents to more than 180 metres, the whale's heart rate dipped to just two beats per minute for fifteen minutes, the lowest recorded heart rate in any animal. It returned to the normal resting rate of thirty beats per minute after surfacing.

For this ploddingly slow rate to deliver enough blood to the 30-tonne body, the researchers found radical adaptations to the main blood vessel leaving the heart. These structural innovations completely changed how blood flowed out from the heart. Replicating these blood-flow patterns allowed Casper to survive on the heart-lung machine and also gave Wales's most notable surgeon, Brian Rees, an extra three years of life despite not having a pulse.

Born in the same small Welsh industrial coal-scarred town as me, Rees was a formidable character. When I first met him as a medical student, his handshake was solid, his voice musical like a male voice choir and his surgical skills legendary. His hands had saved many lives and also scored many tries. The former hooker had won three caps for Wales during the 1967 Five Nations Championship after a successful undergraduate sporting career at Cambridge. In the operating theatre, like on the pitch, he took no bullshit, with colleagues describing him as 'a menace, yet charming, witty and loads of fun'. By 2000, Rees had become the lead cancer clinician at Wales's largest teaching hospital and was awarded an OBE for his services to medicine. He was a well of humanity and passion and left a definite imprint on surgery in the UK, starting the first keyhole surgery training centre. For a surgeon to leave a legacy of fewer stitches is remarkable. When I met Brian Rees twenty years after being his student, the tables were turned. He was very different.

Late one cold, blue winter night, Rees became unwell and was brought to the heart ward at the hospital where I worked. It was my very first night shift as an intensive care consultant and I had hoped for a quiet night. A young doctor called me in a panic, asking for help in managing a complicated patient with heart failure.

'Oh, and by the way, he used to work in the hospital apparently,' they added.

'Ah, interesting. What is his name?' I asked.

'Um, Brian . . . Brian Rees.'

Oh, bloody hell, I thought. This wasn't the first shift I had planned for.

Time carves history into human faces and human hands. Lying in bed, critically unwell, Rees was both the same as I remembered but also very different. The observations shown on the colourful monitor behind his hospital bed were terrible. His blood pressure was in his boots, his heart rate erratic and his oxygen levels dangerously low.

Yet, after introducing myself, his eyes opened with a characteristic twinkle. He stretched out his hand that too had held the hands of thousands of patients over a lifetime of service in medicine. His handshake was as solid as ever. But as I felt his pulse, it was weak and thready. His heart was failing and there was nothing that could be done to fix it. Driving home from hospital the following morning, I knew Rees's days of even watching rugby were limited. He would soon die.

A year later, I gave a talk to the Cardiff Medical Society, the oldest organisation of its kind. My talk formed the basis of this book, telling the audience of mostly retired doctors about my recent visit to Noel Fitzpatrick's innovative veterinary practice during recording of his television series *The Supervet*. The talk was titled 'How Kissing a Frog Can Save Your Life'. I explored early, underdeveloped ideas on how understanding the lives of animals may help treat human disease. I joked how a kangaroo's three vaginas may teach us about human IVF. I told the story you have now read about Ifan, the student who was assaulted, and how a giraffe helped us treat his brain injury. I ended with my newly discovered fact that a whale's heart beats just twice per minute yet can maintain its circulation.

In the nearby bustling pub after the talk, a familiar hand reached out to shake my hand.

'Great talk, boy!' Brian Rees said in that same melodic voice. 'I think I'm like that whale you talked about, apart from the Pink Floyd that is!' he said with a chuckle.

I was flustered and didn't know how to respond.

'Feel this!' he exclaimed as he held out his wrist.

Pressing on his artery as I had done a year ago, I felt something very strange – nothing. No pulse. Nothing.

'I'm only alive thanks to this,' he said, pointing to a battery pack around his shoulder. 'My heart is pumping just like a bloody whale and I'm in extra time!'

As the blue whale dives and its heart rate drops to two beats per minute, its heart squeezes in a different way. The muscle extends its contraction longer, pushing blood for an extended time into the large aorta exiting at the top. The muscular walls of this vessel change their characteristics as the whale's body comes under extreme water pressure at the bottom of the dive. The aorta acts like a big elastic chamber, expanding and contracting with each thumping heartbeat, smoothing each spurting jet of blood into a continuous flow. If the whale had wrists, it too would have no heartbeat, just a continuous hum of blood moving around like Brian's.

Brian Rees still had heart failure with no cure. Yet a mechanical device, implanted deep inside his body weeks after I had met him, deeply unwell in hospital, now continuously pumped blood to his organs. It didn't fix the underlying problem, it couldn't stop him from dying, but this gave him a little extra time. As with the whale, it gave Brian's body just enough blood in a continuous stream, slowly and steadily. So too with Casper, his heart-lung machine was programmed using the latest evidence that showed non-pulsatile, continuous blood flow was better for critically ill patients. Both Brian and Casper survived by using the same strategy as a diving whale does, the same blood-flow patterns. And, like the whale, this allowed life to continue at the very edges of survival.

Sixty years after ships were smashed and lives nearly lost while recording the whale's ECG, we can now stare at its wandering line and apply lessons to human life. Tracing the line with a finger, you will first hit a small hump causing the atria at the top of the heart to contract. After this 'P wave', the next change in the line is the upward 'R wave', causing the powerful bottom ventricular chambers to squeeze. The space between these two waves, known as the PR interval, should vary according to the physical distance between the two parts of the heart in different animals. It was in this space that the mystery lay.

In a mouse, electrical impulses travel over the short millimetre distance in just 30 milliseconds. Humans have a tract that is 5cm long, producing a bigger gap of 200 milliseconds. The bigger the animal, the longer the distance. But, strangely, the size of the gap doesn't always increase in proportion. Instead, this delay is only ten times longer in elephants than in mice, despite the distance being 25,000 times longer. This gave scientists like White and Meijler hints that the function of some heart regions were more complex than simply conducting signals. Instead, they argued, these regions may be control centres. If true, treatments and procedures could be aimed at these critical areas to calm chaotic rhythms in patients like Casper. The gap in the whale's ECG held the key to whether their theory was right.

In the 30-tonne whale, its 180kg heart has a muscular wire connecting the top to the bottom of the heart – 55cm long. Impulses should take 1.5 seconds to travel this distance. Yet the gap on the ECG recorded by Meijler was just 400 milliseconds. A whale's heart is six times larger than an elephant's, thirty times the size of a horse's, yet all have the same PR interval. Meijler and White were right: the area known as the AV node, once considered just a relay station for signals, was so much more. It was a control centre that could be adjusted, tweaked in health and in disease.

Through passion and incremental knowledge passed from whale to White to Frits Meijler and then to fellow electrical heart specialists, in 1981 Dr Melvin Scheinman did something remarkable. Burning tiny areas in this control centre of the heart using hot wires passed though the body, Scheinman cured a retired Californian oil worker's arrhythmias after all other treatments had failed. Soon came new, better and safer procedures. Doctors used this knowledge on Casper's jumping heart, fine-tuning its rhythm using electricity applied through his skin, just like when it was first tried 200 years earlier in 1778 on the cobbled streets of London.

All stories end; some happy, others sad. My teacher, Brian Rees, the rugby star, the surgeon, the pulseless man, did extend his life thanks to a heartbeat like a whale, until 2021. After his death, sports stars, Welsh singers, patients and politicians inked the columns of newspapers paying their compliments to one of the greats.

The story for Casper and his friends is still being written. Hour by hour in February 2011, more and more lives were snatched back from death. First was Casper. His body warmed, his blood oxygen-filled red in colour, and his heart calmed. Every parent in the hospital waiting room screamed with joy when doctors told them Casper had woken up. That day, all seven children who were clinically dead came back to life – the largest number of simultaneous survivors ever described.

But life was just the beginning. The children were moved to live together in a rehabilitation hospital, to heal together. The process was long and tough. Many had signs of brain damage – severe weakness, pain and numbness. The small wooden model of a bike on the shelf behind Casper when I spoke to him was a precious reminder. The first time he was able to move his hands after being paralysed from the accident was to turn the wheel of a hand bike while his dad watched on in the rehabilitation hospital. Slowly, life returned.

Some of the children needed amputations. Research examining how antlers attach to a deer's skull, as in our 20,000-year-old cave painting, may yet help them. Prosthetic limbs implanted into bone are already used in dogs thanks to pioneers like the Supervet, rather than attachments being strapped to flesh. The survivors maintained a special bond, six of the seven finishing school together and going back to a normal life, whatever that means. Tragically, one of the boys, Casper's friend, drowned while swimming on holiday in South America five years later.

Determined not to suffer the same fate, Casper, who couldn't swim at the time of the accident, asked his child-hood sweetheart, a swimming teacher, for help. After returning from a holiday on the Turkish coast, Casper, who died in the water and survived thanks to creatures of the water, is now at home in the water.

'I love swimming now. The water has been good to me,' he tells me with a pirate smile, looking down towards the ground.

THE UNDERLAND

'Into the underland we have long placed that which we fear and wish to lose, and that which we love and wish to save.'

ROBERT MACFARLANE

14

ALONE IN THE MIST

As I opened the door, the room seemed filled with memories rather than sadness. A photo album was being passed from table to table, aged photographs providing a glimpse into a past life well lived. I found an empty seat, feeling clumsy in my own skin as I sat down in an uncomfortable black suit. In my jacket pocket was an order of service from the last funeral I had attended some years before. As I looked around the function room, there were family members I didn't recognise, friends with whom I didn't share any memories, and colleagues that I had not worked with. Why did I feel the need to come at all – to the funeral of someone I had known for just one year? Why did I decide to go to a patient's funeral for the first time since becoming a doctor?

Working on an intensive care unit, death is always a reliable companion. While we strive for life, around one in five of our patients will sadly not survive. While we always care for patients, we also find ourselves caring about them. There are some patients that we can't help but carry along with us. Sometimes it is because they were very young, sometimes because they were very old, sometimes because they said something memorable, and sometimes because they could not speak for themselves.

We are taught in medical school not to treat family or friends except in dire emergencies. But what should we do when those you care for become almost like friends? While working in a big, bustling intensive care unit in Wales as a consultant, I met Roy. I spoke to Roy most weeks for over a year as we tried to help his heart and kidney failure with machines and complex operations. Although then in his seventies, as a younger man he had travelled the world by ship and had plenty of stories to tell.

So did I. I had told him things that normally I would only share with my family. I had told him about events from my past and hopes for the future. I'm not sure why I did this. Roy felt like a stable, familiar feature in an ever-changing mêlée of other patients. He felt like part of the team as well as a patient.

I was there when his wife cried after we broke bad news and helped her smile when Roy eventually pulled through. This wasn't unique to me. Many members of the team had grown even closer to Roy and his family than I. Despite a new heart valve being fitted, it wasn't enough to allow him to live outside of the intensive care unit. And so his life continued inside it. He would spend time with his long-term partner, Lesley. Roy would have good days and bad days. He would even marry Lesley in a wedding held on the unit after a stag party in his bed space. Then Roy died.

Was I an outlier, spending my day off not with my family but with a patient's family? Many would not. Death can be seen as a failure rather than a part of life for many doctors, whose prime industry is delivering a cure. Some argue that a funeral belongs to the family, not the professionals. Emotional distance between doctor and patient may foster better, unattached and less emotive care. However, it can also leave both sides cold. Doctors are not immune from emotions and forcing this façade is hard. What is clear is that we have scant opportunity to share what emotions we do have.

Medical school and national guidelines are designed to answer questions with clear answers. 'How do you treat a heart attack?' the exam paper asks. 'Like this,' we respond with confidence. The humanity that envelops medicine is seldom so simple. Even the most basic ethical questions have complex answers.

When the trays of sandwiches had been cleared away, I waited in line to wish his wife well in the difficult time that would follow. Only then did I realise why I and some of my colleagues had gone to the funeral. Going was a two-way street. I felt part of a community, part of his life more than part of his death. His family also seemed to draw solace from our role that extended beyond his hospital bed. We were not just doctors and nurses – we were people who shared, even wrote, part of their story of life and now were characters in their own story of death. To my surprise, the real reason was not to represent the hospital, or to play my part, but because 'the patient' had become something else. Despite the logical arguments for and against going to his funeral, what compelled me to go was rather simple. Roy had become a friend to me and to many others who had helped care for him. I had simply gone to a funeral for a friend. Are us humans unique in doing this?

Monica Szczupider spoke to me from Hawaii in the months before starting a primatology Ph.D. in New Zealand. She tells me how her Polish immigrant parents made the tough, uncertain journey to the US. Her dad, a factory worker, would relax at home with a nature documentary on TV rather than the Super Bowl, while her mum worked long hours at a grocery shop. Watching *Gorillas in the Mist* one evening curled up on the sofa with her dad, Monica vowed to one day work towards a better understanding with our ape ancestors. And she would, with the opening of a camera's shutter.

Monica's creative outlet in community college was the dark room, which held a special allure. Later, as she travelled the world's continents, her Sony camera would help her tell the stories of those surrounding her, human and animal.

Volunteering in Sanaga-Yong Chimpanzee Rescue Center in Cameroon for six months between university degrees drew her further into the animal community. Her days were spent preparing food for the twenty-five rescued chimps. In her downtime, she taught children in the local village. But it was a sad day in 2008 that changed her life. It was a day that transmitted the ubiquitous nature of loss into the homes of millions.

Around midday, she heard on her radio that Dorothy,

the thirty-year-old elder matriarch of the rescue group, was feared dead. Running in flip-flops towards the shelter, Monica put her head on Dorothy's chest to listen for breathing. She felt her neck for a pulse. Nothing. Nothing. Dorothy had died from heart failure. Although sadly not uncommon in sanctuaries, it was the first chimp Monica had seen die.

Dorothy had not always been the group's respected matriarch. For decades she had been kept in chains, entertainment for tourists after her mum had been shot for bushmeat. After her rescue, adjusting to a new life was tough. Other chimps would bully Dorothy by throwing dirt or using sticks to hit her. Motherhood changed that.

A newly orphaned infant male chimp was introduced to the group. Suddenly, Dorothy took on a protective role, becoming a surrogate mum for four-year-old Bouboule. The next ten years embedded Dorothy as a key member of the group, much loved, respected and valued.

The day after Dorothy died, the sanctuary's founder, Dr Sheri Speede, felt the wider world needed to see Dorothy to help them make sense of what had happened and where Dorothy had gone. People from the local area walked miles to be there. Speede cradled Dorothy's head in her hands as she lay wrapped in a sheet while slowly pushing a cushioned wheelbarrow to where Dorothy would be buried.

Monica's camera shutter blinked open and quickly curled closed. It was perfectly timed to capture the twenty-five other chimps from Dorothy's community who had come running out of the forest, lining up silently to bid their last farewell. They placed their hands on one another's shoulders. What the camera couldn't capture was the noise at that moment – complete silence. This was unheard of when so many primates were together.

Monica is sure this was grief. Silence says so much. The ultimate respect, even in human life, is not a speech or a song, but nothing. Quiet. Speaking to Monica in 2020, she reflected on the funerals of her two close friends who died in their teens and the silence after her dad later died. Sometimes, in grief we become even more alive ourselves.

Millions saw Monica's photo after it won a *National Geographic* competition. Dr Speede later released a book titled *Kindred Beings: What Seventy-Three Chimpanzees Taught Me About Life, Love, and Connection.* The world seemed astonished that animals can have such a human-like reaction to the death of a loved one. I'm surprised that people were surprised.

That simple photo of a silent family can help teach us all that the capacity to love and grieve is not exclusively human. It reinforces the deeply ingrained ways that we can manage to deal with the pain – to touch, to look, to be there, to think, to say goodbye. No wonder I wanted to go to a funeral of a patient. But how radically have our behaviours around death changed in the evolutionary blink of an eye between chimp and human trapped in the concrete jungle?

With echoes of Dunbar's work in primate grooming that we explored in Chapter 2, Monica emphasised the importance of touch during this moment – it was the first time she had seen the apes put their arms around each other in this way. Monica had trained in therapeutic massage herself and hopes modern medicine remembers these simple, yet impactful parts of life that should be used alongside the technological wonders of modern science. In the weeks that follow the loss of a primate family member, their grooming time increases substantially. Yet, working in the most advanced healthcare systems in the world, in the peak of loss in the COVID-19 pandemic, this power of touch was missing. How different death became for humans in the midst of the pandemic.

We live in a blaze of light. Evening comes and then it is night for ever. We can't cure death in ICU. And sometimes the best thing to save is not a life but a good death. The next year and a half showed us all that.

COVID-19 has brought new memories for us all to carry. In a decade's time there will be many patients' faces that I will still carry with me.

I chose intensive care as a medical speciality because I wanted to think as well as to act. Now I realise that above all I just want to communicate: with patients, with families and with colleagues. Communication is healthcare's most valuable and yet most dangerous procedure, verbal dexterity mattering much more than manual. Yet COVID-19 has stolen face-to-face communication with families when they need it the most. Instead, I broke bad news through the twisted cord of a telephone where the power of silence can be mistaken for hanging up.

I know from personal experience that even the sound of your ringtone during a television programme can induce panic when waiting for news of a loved one who is unwell. 'What if it's the hospital?' you think. So now I try to start my phone calls to families with: 'Don't worry, this isn't a bad news call.' Not this time. That would be a lie. It is bad news. The worst.

I begin: 'I'm so sorry to do this over the phone . . .'

The call ends with quiet sobbing.

We promise to hold the patient's hand. To play his favourite song. To tell him that their family loves them. Loved them. Past tense. Because, soon after, they die. We all carry COVID-19, not on our skin but in our heads and in our hearts. It stole our need to be there, to touch, to see, and to walk home with those we love when they die.

I grew up in the Welsh valleys, learning my country's native Gaelic tongue until I was sixteen years old. I am embarrassed that although I can sing the national anthem at international rugby matches and have a strong Welsh accent, I cannot speak Welsh. Luckily, the foreign language of modern medicine came easier when I started at medical school. A large part of my training was becoming fluent in an age-old language I would never speak outside the hospital. Today I understand lost words from ancient Greece and I am fluent in Latin, so long as the conversation is only about anatomy. This is perhaps why communicating on difficult topics can be hard and the cause of so many patient or family complaints. When breaking bad news, your mind works in one language while your mouth talks another. I feel like there are two singing birds on my shoulders, one speaking in medicine, one in human.

Dorothy was not the first chimp to show us the ingrained cultural practices around death. Many have described how, after a death, chimps pace around, sniff, touch and rearrange bodies into different positions. Mothers often carry their dead young around for weeks or months, continuing to care, protect and communicate with their child. They sometimes groom them for days until they are decayed and no longer recognisable.

Baboons reach out for help from their friends after a death. Dr Anne Engh, a researcher at the University of Pennsylvania's Department of Biology, describes how a baboon named Sylvia needed help from her friends after her daughter was killed by a lion. Baboons respond to bereavement in similar ways to humans, levels of stress hormones rising including cortisol. But they can lower these through increased social contact, expanding their grooming network and grooming time.

'Like humans, baboons seem to rely on friendly relationships to help them cope with stressful situations,' she says.

These behaviours are not restricted to primates. Elephants live in rich communities with discrete cultures. They self-medicate with plants, protect humans and animals, and even make art. Incredibly, elephants paint. An elephant named Karishma is a keen painter at a zoo in Dunstable, England, with her paintings shown as part of the zoo's Elephant Appreciation Weekend every year.

After the death of a key member of a South African elephant group, researcher Martin Meredith described in his book a typical death ritual:

'The entire family of a dead matriarch, including her young calf, were all gently touching her body with their trunks, trying to lift her. The elephant herd were all rumbling loudly. The calf was observed to be weeping and made sounds that sounded like a scream, but then the entire herd fell incredibly silent. They then began to throw leaves and dirt over the body and broke off tree branches to cover her. They spent the next two days quietly standing over her body. They sometimes had to leave to get water or food, but they would always return.'

When finding a dead elephant, groups will touch the bones or body gently with their trunks. Staying very quiet, they cover the body with leaves and grass. Families have been known to stay with dead family members for weeks after death, often revisiting grave sites in cycles. In Kenya, an elephant that trampled a human mother and child stopped to bury them.

In the air, too, animals say goodbye. Magpies are the only non-mammal who can recognise themselves in a mirror. Perhaps linked to this sense of self and others, Dr Marc Bekoff, from the University of Colorado, says that magpies 'feel grief and hold funerals'. After observing the death of a magpie within a family of four, he describes how: 'One approached the corpse, gently pecked at it, just as an elephant would nose the carcass of another elephant, and stepped back. Another magpie did the same thing.'

He goes on to say: 'Next, one of the magpies flew off, brought back some grass and laid it by the corpse. Another magpie did the same. Then all four stood vigil for a few seconds and one by one flew off.'

Even under the sea, death does not go by in silence. Sea lions, dolphins and seals will cry out for days over the loss of a baby. Even when stillborn, mothers will remain close to the child for days, cuddling, nuzzling and calling. In July 2018, a mother orca named Tahlequah carried her dead infant for seventeen days, pushing it with her nose as she travelled thousands of miles.

What do these animal practices tell us about human death and how our increasing distance between the dead and the living may affect grief?

Rhian Burke knows only too well these visceral feelings of loss. Her son, George, died suddenly from severe infection when he was just one year, one week and one day old. The clinically clean, efficient emergency department had nowhere to put George, nowhere for the family to touch him, to spend time with him, nothing to wrap him in. Rhian instead followed behind as a nurse carried her dead son down corridors, past onlookers, to a closed children's ward with cartoon characters on the walls where she could spend time with George. Racked with grief, her husband Paul killed himself by jumping from a local bridge five days later.

The Western world is in an epidemic of death denial. Even after someone has died. In her book *Smoke Gets in Your Eyes*, mortician Caitlin Doughty describes the invasive and often unnecessary funeral practices common today, such as ultra-rapid corpse removal from homes, extreme embalming techniques and exploitative unnatural viewing ceremonies.

Chimps, elephants, seals and even birds have shown us that time spent with those you love after death is a golden thread sewn through loss over millions of years. Home used to be where the corpse was, Doughty says. Now they lie in a refrigerated, commercial multinational industrial unit with a glossy brochure. The home was where support networks would congregate, where help from a friend was offered and taken. Where your mum or dad or child would stay for sometimes days after they had died. Even in intensive care, it is not unusual for husbands and wives, mothers and fathers, to get into bed with their loved one after they have died. Just to hold them. Just to be there.

And these olden cross-species rituals, which are hard to understand outside of the dark lens of grief, may help us deal with loss. Studies show that spending time with the dead may reduce the duration and severity of grief.

As Rhian sat at home, surrounded by flowers and photos of her two boys who had died in less than a week, she did something truly remarkable. She used her grief to help others.

Rather than allow these unimaginable events to destroy her, Rhian founded the charity 2wish, which funds thoughtful family rooms in hospitals, ideally designed for breaking bad news, complete with bereavement boxes that allow lasting memories to be made from handprints and hair cuttings after a sudden death. She didn't want another parent to walk down corridors with their child in their arms. When I sit in our relatives' room today, it is thanks to Rhian's strength that families have a better experience than she once had. Working in the dark means you see everything. My good days bring happiness, my bad ones experience and gratefulness.

The charity's mascot is an elephant.

15

HAPPY 392ND BIRTHDAY

It could have burnt the whole retirement home to the ground. Thankfully, the cake wasn't big enough to hold all 117 candles.

Sister André is Europe's oldest person. She has been there and done that – the First World War, the Russian Revolution, the invention of the television, the Second World War, the polio vaccine, colour television, the vote for women, the 1918 flu pandemic, the Great Depression and now the COVID-19 pandemic.

Her 117th birthday lunch in February 2021 in the French city of Toulon included port wine, followed by foie gras with hot figs, roasted capon with mushrooms and sweet potatoes as a main course, followed by a two-cheese platter and a glass of red wine. To finish, a raspberry and peach flavoured baked Alaska with a glass of Champagne. No cocktail-sticked sausages in sight.

Sister André claims her daily red wine is her secret to longevity and the reason she survived COVID-19 after the infection killed ten of her younger friends at her retirement home. But today, on her 117th birthday, she is in 'great shape and really happy'.

Born in 1904 in a small southern French town, she worked as a governess in Marseille then as a tutor in Paris. Turning to God through a Catholic conversion at age nineteen, she then turned to medicine at the age of twenty-five, working as a nurse caring for the elderly and orphaned children. What might be considered later in life, but was really only one-third of the way through, at forty she changed her name from Lucile Randon to Sister André following her religious calling, becoming a nun. André was the name of her late brother.

When Sister André was found to have COVID-19, she told a reporter: 'I wasn't scared because I wasn't scared of dying. When you've been an adolescent during a pandemic that killed tens of millions, and seen the horrors of two world wars, you do put things into perspective.'

When asked about the current pandemic, she says simply: 'It will come and go.'

Despite her tenacity, every day Sister André steps closer to the upper end of human lifespan: 122 years. While graphs show increasing life expectancy as centuries roll by, this figure is distorted by improvements in infant mortality rates. The true upper end of human longevity has changed remarkably little over generations despite multivitamins, red wine and hair transplants.

If I'm honest, I'm also not afraid of dying, but am afraid of living too fast or too slow. Sister André reminds us that death lasts only minutes but life lasts for ever. In the end, we are all just walking each other home. But why do we die? Do we have to?

Like Sister André, Harriet has also lived through a lot – the First World War, the Russian Revolution, the television, the Second World War, the polio vaccine, colour television, the vote for women, the 1918 flu pandemic and the Great Depression. Abraham Lincoln was assassinated when she was thirty-five years old. Harriet was already eighty-two when, in 1912, the *Titanic* sank. She also lived through an Englishman called Charles Darwin arriving at her home, packing her in a box and sailing with her to Australia. Because Harriet is a giant Galápagos tortoise.

Harriet is reported to have been one of three giant tortoises taken from the Galápagos Islands. She was just five years old and no bigger than a dinner plate when she was first taken to Britain then on to Australia. Harriet was initially named Harry, after Harry Oakman, the creator of the zoo at the Brisbane Botanic Gardens, after a minor gender mix-up. She died in 2006, aged 176, after becoming a celebrity in a zoo owned by the late Steve Irwin. Harriet had used no beauty creams or preservatives, drunk no red wine and taken no multivitamins, yet beat her human counterparts hands down.

Harriet wasn't even the oldest ever tortoise. Guinness World Records lists 188-year-old Tui Malila, a Madagascan tortoise presented to Tonga's royal family by British explorer Captain James Cook in the 1770s, as the oldest.

Tortoises are not the only animals that outlive us. The Greenland shark lives for a minimum of 272 years, with some swimming around 392 years ago, when St Peter's Basilica in the Vatican had just been completed and Galileo had just arrived in Rome for his trial before the Inquisition. The New Zealand tuatara lizard lives for more than a hundred years and the immortal jellyfish continuously cycles between child and adult phases, riding around the world on the bottom of ships. It can live for ever. Who needs unicorns and fairies when we have creatures like this?

Understanding how and why these extreme feats of longevity are possible is not just important for Hollywood actors maxed out on vitamin infusions and stem cell injections. A better grasp of longevity may help humans live within standard lifespans but with an improved quality of life. Many chronic illnesses that erode our sunset years are due to the slow footsteps towards our mortality limits. Rates of cancer, arthritis and dementia all increase dramatically the closer we step to our end. So, understanding how to better manage or even bypass ageing mechanisms will help us not cure death but rather improve life. Few people want 392 candles on their birthday cake like the Greenland shark, but many want to do the conga around the street as they mark their centenary. One strange, blind creature from Africa could help make this possible – the naked mole rat.

A round, fleshy circular nose like a shaved arsehole. Sticking out from the middle of its face, two yellowed long teeth with wiry whiskers sprouting all around. Two small eyes fixed on to the side of its face with tiny folded ears, all covered in loose, pink, piglet-like skin. This is Joe, from the underground tropical grasslands of East Africa. Joe has looked exactly the same since he was born in 1982, even though he's got a big birthday coming up – the big 4-0! Like a character in a superhero video, Joe hardly ages, doesn't feel pain and will not get cancer. He won't win any beauty contests but may help us live for ever.

Similar-sized mammals like mice live to around four years of age. Naked mole rats should live to six, yet often reach thirty years, remaining fertile until the end. That is the equivalent of humans having a baby aged 300. Most strikingly, the naked mole rat breaks a fundamental law of ageing, known as Gompertz law. It is named after the British mathematician Benjamin Gompertz, who in 1825 found that the risk of death in mammals rises exponentially with age. In humans, the risk of death doubles every eight years. Yet, after the naked mole rat reaches sexual maturity, its chances of dying remain completely flat at 1 in 10,000 for the rest of their lives.

Naked mole rats do age and do get sick, but these processes are super slow. While my bones have started to thin
compared with when I was in my thirties, the mole rat's
bones remain solid. They also don't put on weight as they
age, but most surprising is what happens to their blood
vessels – nothing.

'Every measure that we've looked at in heart function
is unchanged from six months to twenty-four years,' says
Rochelle Buffenstein, who has studied naked mole rats
since the 1980s and now works for Google's anti-ageing
Calico Labs. Their blood vessels do not harden, do not
accumulate fatty deposits and their hearts continue to efficiently squeeze.

It is important not to over-interpret and over-apply these
data. Naked mole rats are very strange mammals, almost
entirely cold-blooded with low metabolic rates. Direct
application of these findings to humans must be treated with
extreme caution. However, these studies do suggest that
the natural slip to chronic disease in life is optional. Studies
have shown excellent DNA repair mechanisms in naked
mole rats along with high levels of chaperone molecules,
which keep proteins folding correctly. It is these errors of
DNA repair and folding that ultimately results in cancer.
The naked mole rat also has genes that recognise when cells
are overcrowded, an early hallmark of cancer, and prevent
further cell divisions. These point to new mechanisms that
cancer drugs could target, preventative treatments that

could be applied and how our understanding of ageing could improve the lives of patients.

🐀

Taken together, scientists now think the naked mole rat lives 'its life in pulses',* having periods of high activity with longer downtimes during which they are almost in a state of suspended animation. They live in large colonies of up to 300, often in burrows deep underground with low levels of oxygen. This may explain their extreme resistance to low oxygen levels, much like what happens in humans having a stroke or heart attack. Naked mole rats can survive at least five hours in air containing only 5 per cent oxygen, which is very different to my patients in my ICU who can develop brain injuries after only minutes exposed to low oxygen levels. They can even cope with zero oxygen for a whopping eighteen minutes. Although their hearts nearly stop and they lose consciousness, naked mole rats recover completely when exposed to normal air.

One reason this is possible is by switching from a normal metabolic pathway using glucose as a fuel to this biological downtime using instead fructose, the sugar found in fruits. Drugs exploiting these novel pathways in human diseases like heart attacks and strokes are now being studied. Mole rats rarely die from spontaneous disease like other animals, but rather trauma or infection.

---

* A quote from Stan Braude, Ph.D., lecturer in biology in Arts & Sciences at Washington University in St Louis in a press release titled 'Ugly duckling mole rats might hold key to longevity' by Erin Fults, 4 October 2007.

Although this research is startling and possibly life-changing, there is one question that still needs to be asked: 'Is this okay?' While half a million children die from simple diarrhoea every year, we are trying to eke out every last year of life like toothpaste from a rolled-up tube. We spend up to £6,000 a day on frail patients in some intensive care units while this amount could save 100 years of children's lives from malaria by buying 2,000 mosquito nets. Three billion dollars' worth of Botox is sold globally per year, yet 50 per cent of the estimated 100 million people who need insulin globally can't afford it. The World Health Organization estimates that $1 billion is spent on AIDS research and $0.5 billion trying to beat malaria. This is eclipsed by the estimated $2 billion spent worldwide on surgical procedures addressing male pattern baldness when a hat would suffice. Now a commercial company, Libella Gene Therapeutics, is charging volunteers $1 million for gene therapy that it claims can reverse ageing by up to twenty years. And anyway, do you really want to live for ever?

Kneeling on the polished stone floor, Nareerat and her husband Sahatorn hug a little girl's white dress tight to their chests. They chant Buddhist prayers while their reflections bounce off a highly polished metal vat. Inside is their two-year-old daughter's frozen brain.

Einz was first diagnosed with brain cancer just a few months earlier in her home city of Bangkok. Her dad, a laser scientist, had been desperately researching novel treatments for her cancer. But after ten operations, twelve rounds of chemotherapy and twenty of radiotherapy, there was no hope left.

While in Bali, I met the award-winning journalist and filmmaker Pailin Wedel. Over hot soup and noodles, she told me about her documentary, Hope Frozen, that followed the family's remarkable decision to freeze their daughter's brain, hoping one day that she could again live.

After dying in Bangkok, her mum held her hand and said: 'Come back one day and be my daughter again. Mummy loves you so much.' Her body was then rapidly cooled before being transported to Arizona, where her brain was removed and stored at -196°C using liquid nitrogen.

The family hope that Einz can be resuscitated in the future when a cure for her disease has been discovered. Einz now 'lives' frozen in time at the life-extension company Alcor's headquarters in Arizona, one of the hottest states in America. She is the youngest person ever to be preserved using this technology. Einz's brother, Matrix, is now pursuing a career in science hoping to find a way of bringing back his sister sometime in the future.

With our naked ape's ability to go to the Moon, venture to Mars and understand string theory, perhaps we will soon be able to consign death entirely to the history books. Would life be better if we didn't die? Sixteen hundred miles away from Einz's frozen brain in Arizona, a tiny squirrel-like creature found in the Canadian wilderness may just help Matrix save his sister.

Indigenous people have long lived in the high mountains and dense forests of the Rocky Mountains, getting by through hunting bison, fishing and trapping. What is now called Banff National Park was a sacred place where medicines were gathered and healing ceremonies conducted in hot springs. Yet underground, a tiny creature lived without the fire that kept these people warm, without the bearskins and without even needing to find food for much of the year. The high-pitched trill of the yellow-bellied marmot would only be heard for a third of the year because for the other two-thirds it would be asleep. Almost frozen, entirely still.

The marmot is marvellous for what it doesn't do. For eight months a year it hibernates through tough winters in Canada and other mountain regions from the Himalayas to the Alps. This full-body shutdown affects organs from the heart, slowing from a normal 120 to just three to four beats per minute, to the liver making glucose from its large stores of glycogen. Amazingly, a marmot's blood pressure stays normal despite the slow heartbeat thanks to the way its blood vessels constrict. Their breathing also slows to just two breaths a minute and their temperature dips as low as 5°C. Remarkably, during hibernation a marmot's genetic clock stops, with ageing seemingly frozen in time. To anyone who has been trapped in a winter lodge on a snowy day with little to do other than drink hot chocolate and eat fondue, just as incredible is the marmot's lack of appetite. A chemical messenger called AICAR turns off the desire to eat and stops areas of the brain associated with obesity in humans from being active.

Although this may lend positivity to the notion of a deep freeze being possible to extend a human lifetime, even the 5-degree temperature over eight months that marmots survive can't be compared with Einz's tank in Arizona. But maybe amphibians can help.

Even by Canadian standards of cold, the adaptations needed to survive an Alaskan winter are extreme. The Wim Hof of these conditions is the wood frog. With temperatures above the Arctic Circle as low as -35°C, simply slowing down its heartbeat would not be enough. At these temperatures, diesel freezes and so there is little hope for blood to keep flowing around the body normally. But the frog has a trick – anti-freeze.

Before hibernation, wood frogs raise the levels of glucose in their bodies so high that it acts as a natural anti-freeze. Like adding grit to roads, high sugar levels decrease the freezing point of liquids, preventing ice crystals from forming in organs. This allows tissues to freeze in a gradual, controlled manner and then to thaw out safely when warmer months arrive. But as the marmot can't compete with the wood frog, the frog can't compete with the Siberian salamander.

The Russian port of Magadan has had a troubled history after being used as a transit centre in the 1930s for political prisoners to forced labour camps. Deep underfoot, while soldiers marched and prisoners perished, a Siberian salamander became stuck in a tree stump hibernation site. After filling with water, the gaps in the stump formed a wedge of ice that stayed frozen even during the summer months. This became the home for that salamander. Long after the prisoners were freed, the Soviet Union crumbled and forced labour was replaced by rafting tourists, a team at Magadan's Institute for Biological Problems of the North found the trapped salamander. It had been there for ninety years.

This was not the oldest specimen they have found. Some had been extracted 14 metres deep in the permafrost, deposited in the Pleistocene age more than 12,000 years ago. The team had already shown salamanders could survive in temperatures as low as -50°C. But this was the first salamander to come back to life after ninety long frozen years. The team described how they placed it into a bucket of cold water to help it very gradually thaw. First the ice on the outside melted, and then, many hours later, it started swimming once again. It had lived through Hope Frozen.

The key to this astonishing survival was the slow, steady freeze. Salamanders can die from sudden frost conditions.

Like the wood frog, they need time to adapt and produce another 'anti-freeze' chemical. Stronger than high sugar levels, salamanders use anti-freeze chemicals more like that used in the cars that drive around the Siberian wilderness. Their enormous liver produces alcohol compounds, like glycerol, which prevent ice crystals from damaging organs. With the glycerol anti-freeze spreading throughout a salamander's body, researchers found that although some crystals of ice form under the skin, the main tissues remained elastic and appeared healthy. Their liver, the largest in proportion to body size of any vertebrate, also is the powerhouse providing a constant energy source, converting stores of glycogen into energy during the long freeze.

The chances of Einz coming back to life like the Siberian salamander are vanishingly rare. But these extreme winter survivalists can teach us lessons to be used in many other areas of medicine. How tissues are protected despite extreme cold temperatures may lead to novel ways to preserve the function of organs destined for transplantation. The slow, steady, safe freeze rates have been replicated in patients undergoing deep hypothermic cardiac arrest – where the heart and brain shuts down for a limited period during high-risk operations on blood vessels of the brain and heart. And the use of anti-freeze compounds derived from alcohols may hint at new ways to further the survival of humans against the odds, maybe even in future cases like Einz.

If you did wake up after a 100-year-long cold sleep, what would you be thinking? Your body may survive, but would your mind? We are already in a pandemic of mental health struggles paired with high levels of drug misuse. Can animals teach us how to keep our minds clear in the rattling pace of present and future extended human life?

16

CRACKED BUT NOT BROKEN

Life-extension companies offering to cryopreserve your brain for eternity seldom discuss the psychological aspects of living for ever. Even if modern medicine could stop joints from creaking and skin from sagging, our minds may crack. After your mum and dad, your son and daughter, your neighbours, your friends and your enemies have all died, life could feel like solitary confinement.

Even without an extra lifetime, one in four of us struggle with our mental health each year. Suicide is the leading cause of death for women and men in their prime between twenty and thirty-five years old in the UK. Perhaps we should worry less about cancer killing us and more about us killing us. Is this unique to our species? Are Homo sapiens designed to cry? Perhaps this is the price we must pay for human intelligence and creativity and love. Can animals help dry our tears?

The moment Kevin jumped headfirst from the bridge, he

no longer wanted to die. But it was too late. He plummeted from the brick-red Golden Gate Bridge, striking the concrete-like water at 75mph after falling the equivalent of twenty-five storeys.

Kevin's suicide journey started long before he was even born. Found alone on a stained mattress in a San Francisco slum just a few months old, his parents' subsequent drug addiction after Kevin was placed in care ended only after their early deaths. Even with loving adopted parents, Kevin struggled with his thoughts after turning seventeen. Kevin's high school drama teacher and role model shot himself in the head. Seven months later, on 25 September 2000, death seemed the only way to silence the voices that nineteen-year-old Kevin kept hearing as part of his bipolar disorder.

Five thousand miles away, ten-year-old Hendrix also jumped from a bridge. The golden retriever joined 500 other dogs who had leapt over the stone-cold edge of Overtoun Bridge, nuzzled in the green countryside of rural Scotland. It was nicknamed Dog Suicide Bridge.

What do these stories have in common? Why do humans hurt themselves by using drugs, avoiding sleep and killing themselves? How can animals help us heal the scars that blister not on our skin, but in our hearts and in our heads? Could Hendrix help Kevin? And how did both animals survive when they should have died?

My dog, Chester, runs towards the noise, his long, thin tongue hanging from the side of his mouth, flapping in the air. His red fur is pushed back over his face from the speed he runs towards the footsteps on our gravelled driveway. He launches himself on to the bag-laden human, his tail like a windscreen wiper on the highest setting. He licks their face, grabs on to their leg with his curly paws. No one watching this scene could deny that Chester is happy. He is absolutely ecstatic. And all because my daughter has come home from school, as she does every weekday.

We don't need an MRI scan to show that dogs experience joy. But those scans show that when dogs are reunited with their human guardians, they have elevated brain activity in the same regions that process joy in humans. This has been replicated in most mammals, from primates to the tiny shrew. But does sadness come as an unwelcome passenger along with joy? If so, can animals help us understand and manage human depression?

John Daniel was different from other boys his age. By three, he had his own bedroom, was potty trained, went to school, made his own bed and even did the washing-up. He loved being driven around his small English village in a blood-red convertible car. Life had been tough since his parents were shot in Africa shortly after John Daniel was born. But thirty-year-old Alyce Cunningham had come to his rescue, raising John Daniel as her own between a house in London's Sloane Street and her countryside home in Gloucestershire.

Beautifully mannered, John Daniel enjoyed many typical English rituals, from dinner parties with Alyce's friends to cream tea on a Sunday. He also enjoyed a tot of whisky in the evenings and drinking cold cider on the village green outside the Old Crown pub in Uley. This toddler could handle his drink. Because John Daniel was a 100kg lowland African gorilla.

By 1921, at four years old, John Daniel had become too big to be safely cared for at home. Alyce reluctantly sold him to an American, who promised to give him a better life. Instead, John Daniel toured with the famous Barnum circus, although he didn't make it into the cast list of Hugh Jackman's *The Greatest Showman*. Desperately homesick, missing Alyce and his friends, John Daniel's health quickly went downhill. His new owners wrote to Alyce saying: 'John Daniel pining and grieving for you. Can you not come at once?'

Alyce caught the first ship from Liverpool to New York. Midway, she had the news that John Daniel had died, from grief.

There is a risk of anthropomorphising cases of apparent animal depression and suicide. Peering into the emotional lives of animals may be beyond human comprehension. How can we ever appreciate a dolphin's feelings when hearing the sonar ping from a long-lost child? What is it like for bees to see flowers in glorious ultraviolet light or for an octopus to change colour when scared?

Despite these shortcomings, we should acknowledge some similarities. Humans, like other social animals, are not designed to be solitary. We evolved in tribes, needing to interact, to coexist and to communicate. The absence of these meaningful social connections, snatched away from many primates in captivity, triggers the same processes as physical trauma and critical illness in humans. Desmond Morris's book *The Human Zoo* recognised the enormous wrenching transition from our past lives on the tribal savannah to the present squashed existences of millions by saying:

'The city is not a concrete jungle, it is a human zoo.'

What can we learn from animals to help ease our transition from the plains of Africa to the human zoo? If Chester stopped his joyful welcome homes, we may take him to the vet, worried about depression. They would ask about Chester's diet, how much exercise he was having and who he spent time with during the day while we were all at work. The vet's prescription pad would remain the last resort only after modification of Chester's environment. Historically, human doctors haven't asked these questions despite the 'biopsychosocial model' being a standard part of medical training since the 1970s.

The truth is, modifying these messy parts of life is hard. As the author of *The Happy Brain*, Dr Dean Burnett, says: 'Perhaps reliance on antidepressants is due to incredible pressures of time, money and workload on medical professionals, and alternative treatments require many hours of one-on-one interaction with trained experts, rather than swallowing a few capsules a week?'

This shouldn't diminish the organic, biological, neurotransmitter basis for many serious mental health disorders, including Kevin's. Clearly, there are cases where the drugs and medical interventions are essential alongside or instead of environment changes. So too perhaps in animals, where the use of antidepressants has increased over the last ten years with eight out of ten vets prescribing the human drug Prozac to dogs.

Thankfully, things are changing in human medicine through innovations that encourage human doctors to act more like vets. GPs are now encouraged to use social prescribing, where a gym membership, an art class or even a comedy gig can be written on a prescription pad rather than a drug. Just like the vet asking about Chester's diet, exercise and social life, encouraging humanity is now at the centre of managing patients' mood disorders. This social prescribing overcomes time constraints and barriers, outsourcing the one-on-one needs of patients to where humans belong – the community, their tribe, the outside world. It is a return to human. This change is back towards the way mood disorders in animals have long been treated by vets and their human guardians.

The best mood tonic may not be a drug or even social prescribing but another life – an animal's. Loneliness is a major killer of the elderly, ahead of cancer and heart disease. The lonely's chances of dying early are ten times that of the socially connected. Loneliness damages health as much as smoking fifteen cigarettes a day and is a stronger risk factor than obesity. Reattaching social connections to others through clubs, hobbies or groups can help. But so may a cat, a dog or even a goat.

Racehorse owners have long used goats as companion animals to calm a horse's nerves and anxiety before an important race. Rivals would sometimes unsettle horses by stealing their companion, hence the phrase 'got your goat'. The American racehorse Eldaafer was so attached to his companion goat, Google, that he became inconsolable before an important race in Kentucky after Google was left at his home stables. The goat was quickly flown to be reunited with Eldaafer who went on to win a major $100,000 race. To prevent similar problems, Eldaafer now has a second companion goat called Yahoo.

Companion animals are increasingly used by humans to manage a range of conditions from epilepsy to chronic pain. This is a difficult area to study and research gaps remain. However, studies have shown many positive impacts of companion animal use on physical, psychological and social health. This is especially true in neurodevelopmental disorders such as autism, depression, rehabilitation and even dementia.

In my intensive care unit, the week's highlight is a visit

from our newest staff member, Maggie. The nine-year-old golden retriever does her own ward round, seeing critically ill patients, their relatives and the tired staff caring for them. I often think Maggie does far more good on her morning walk than my morning ward round. On Maggie's first visit, neurology specialists were amazed when a patient with a major stroke moved their right hand to stroke her soft fur. Despite weeks of intensive rehabilitation, this was the first time the patient had been able to move their hand. Hair of the dog may have a scientific basis after all, not for curing hangovers but supporting critically ill patients. A stroke helped treat a stroke.

In April 1970, American animal rights activist and former animal trainer Ric O'Barry visited Kathy the dolphin at the Miami Seaquarium. Kathy filled my childhood Sunday afternoons as the main character in the television show *Flipper*. She was the intelligent dolphin who helped solve local crimes like an underwater version of Lassie. O'Barry had originally captured Kathy and trained her for the show. Sadly, the dolphin's retirement was spent alone in a small concrete tank, very damaging for such a social animal. O'Barry claims Kathy swam into his arms after their reunion before sinking to the bottom of the tank. She refused to resurface, drowning herself.

Kevin believed the voices telling him he needed to die. The seventh version of his suicide note simply read: 'I don't want to be here anymore. To my best friend. You'll find another best friend.' But understanding the motivations of Kathy the dolphin or Hendrix the dog, who leapt from the Scottish bridge, is more difficult.

Animals in captivity or stressful situations clearly show self-destructive behaviour. However, many urban legends such as mass suicide in lemmings are now known to be side effects of severe environmental conditions. For lemmings, mass death occurs when dense populations immigrate at the same time. Many experts in animal behaviour stress that animal suicide is simply a question we cannot answer. While we can examine behaviour, we cannot infer intention. Even more fundamentally, to mean to die, you must first know you are alive. This is very difficult to prove in animals, with few exceptions.

In some cases of apparent animal suicide, intention can be entirely discounted. The parasitic worm Spinochordodes tellinii uses grasshoppers as a host. When fully grown, the worm alters the insects' behaviour, causing them to leap to an early death, allowing the worm to continue its reproduction cycle in water. Kevin was no grasshopper but researchers in Denmark have studied 45,000 women to better understand how parasitic infection may affect human mood.

Toxoplasma gondii, an ancient infection likely first transmitted to humans by domesticated cats in Egypt around 4000 BC, is commonly transmitted from mother to baby during childbirth. Infected women were over 50 per cent more likely to attempt suicide and twice as likely to succeed than those without toxoplasma infection. This risk was increased further with higher levels of parasitism and present even in women with no history of mental illness. Proving causation is very difficult – poor mental health may even increase susceptibility to infections like toxoplasma. However, animals like the grasshopper have led to this important new field of research. What lives inside us may affect the way we think and behave, live and die.

Salvador Dali once said: 'I don't do drugs. I am drugs.' He may have been right. Some claim drugs that are today illegal have helped make us who we are. The American mystic Terence McKenna coined the term 'stoned ape', arguing that psychedelic mushrooms were an evolutionary catalyst for language, imagination, arts, religion, philosophy, science and human culture. The 20,000-year-old deer cave art that started our journey may have been scratched by a stoned Welsh ape.

Redemption through drugs certainly didn't happen for Kevin, whose life was scarred by them. Although his parents didn't use drugs until after he was born, as many as one in forty pregnant women use addictive substances during pregnancy, resulting in drug-addicted babies. Is this unique to humans? Are there alcoholic animals and meth-addicted mammals? And how can understanding drug-taking in animals help humans like Kevin?

I woke with a terrible hangover a week after recovering

from COVID-19. The loss of taste and smell that I had been left with inspired my friends to invent a new game. Could they buy a drink from the well-stocked spirit bar that I could actually taste? Despite the increasingly bizarre colours and flavours of the shots, I could taste nothing. Not even the 63 per cent proof rum. The night ended with laughter, nuts and a sing-along. The morning felt very different.

I experienced first-hand how alcohol allows humans to borrow happiness from tomorrow. Yet this popular poison is ingrained on our ape brain. Studies have shown that one in five monkeys prefer a cocktail of alcohol mixed with sugar water over sugar water alone. Younger monkeys are more likely to drink than older individuals, with most drinking done by teenagers. Dr Robert Dudley proposed the 'Drunken Monkey' hypothesis, explaining primates' love of this poison by the higher calories in fermented foods. Our attraction to alcohol may go back more than 45 million years to the origin of fruit-eating monkeys. Evolution may have selected for pissed primates.

Alcohol is just a gateway drug even in the animal kingdom. Deep in the cragged Canadian Rocky Mountains, bighorn sheep deviate by miles from their foraging territory to satisfy their addiction to hallucinogenic lichen. They grind their teeth to the gums to get their fix by scraping the drug from frozen boulders. In 2009, Tasmanian attorney general Lara Giddings reported that wallabies were causing major problems for crop security. They were 'entering poppy fields, getting as high as a kite and going around in circles'. Who needs aliens when mashed marsupials cause crop circles thanks to their love of opium? Cows eat toxic locoweed that makes them high. Like Kevin's first few hours of life, these toxins then pass to their calves who are born as addicts. Even my pet cat, Elsa, is a feline junkie. Seventy per cent of cats respond strongly to nepetalactone, known by its street name 'catnip'. Produced by plants as a sex pheromone, this LSD-like drug changes cats' behaviour, causing them to roll around, meow or growl, become hyperactive or aggressive, rub themselves and eventually pass out. Jaguars, the domestic cat's distant cousin, seek out similar plants containing psychedelic DMT compounds. Animals seem to love drugs.

Rob Pilley didn't mean to get high. He just wanted to eat his carrots. Sadly, his foraged roots were actually wild hemlock, leading to wild hallucinations and a near-death experience. A few years earlier, Rob had captured another inquisitive animal, but one that did mean to get high.

From an early age, Rob's dad told stories of his grandmother taming wild cobras during India's monsoon seasons. His childhood home was awash with exotic animals, from poisonous frogs to green lizards. This nature immersion inspired Rob to study zoology before joining a world-leading team filming wildlife in their natural habitats using cameras disguised as animals.

In Mozambique in 2014, Rob spent hours watching one of his favourite animals, the bottlenose dolphin. Using a plastic turtle and rubber puffer fish with hidden cameras, Rob entered the dolphins' underwater world. The morning after staying up late drinking cold beers with friends, the ocean's bobbing combined with a hangover proved a tricky combination. Soon Rob would capture wild dolphins socialising with their own friends with help from a different, more dangerous drug than hemlock or alcohol.

A pod of teenage dolphins noticed a solitary poisonous puffer fish swimming by. Nudging it with their noses, they started to gently pass the deadly creature back and forth. These fish contain tetrodotoxin, a toxin 120,000 times more deadly than cocaine. It is hundreds of times more lethal than venom from the cobras his grandmother had befriended. It is even more potent than VX nerve gas and ricin. Tetrodotoxin is quite literally one of the most toxic compounds known to man.

Yet Rob saw these teenagers 'chewing the puffer and gently passing it round. They began acting most peculiarly, hanging around with their noses at the surface as if fascinated by their own reflection.'

After studying this behaviour with experts, the team came to one conclusion – the dolphins were purposefully getting high using a carefully administered amount of poison. Without any culinary training, the dolphins were more skilled than Japanese fugu chefs, who would train for years to serve adventurous diners raw puffer fish with just enough poison to make their lips tingle without causing death. This was the first time this drug-taking behaviour had been described in dolphins.

Before you rush to the pub or a café in Amsterdam, using your animal instincts as an excuse for debauchery, drugs should remind us of the importance of social connection. Canadian psychologist Dr Bruce Alexander's 1970 'Rat Park' experiment echoes the lonely, concrete jungle syndrome that afflicts many humans today. Researchers had shown that rats placed alone in a cage with two water bottles, one filled with water and the other with heroin, would continually drink from the drug bottles. They only stopped when they overdosed and died. Dr Alexander showed that when rats were free to roam, play, socialise and reproduce with others, things changed. The rats stopped dying. Most instead drank from the plain water bottle, and even those who did dabble in drugs used them for only short periods, in a safe, controlled manner without overdosing.

Taken together with our deeply ingrained drug-seeking behaviour, animals can show us health policies that could help tackle today's drug pandemic. The simple and wholesome 'Just say no' strategy is doomed to fail when empty human relationships are combined with in-built selection and track marks stretching back millions of years. Instead, learning lessons from dolphins, apes and rats should encourage harm-reduction approaches. Safe drug consumption rooms have already prevented 230 drug deaths in one Canadian state in just twenty months, with 800 overdoses managed without a single death in one Danish centre.

This is not to admit defeat or endorse drug use, but

rather to embrace human behaviour and human history to temper harms. We didn't ban cars when road traffic deaths increased, we promoted seat belts. Taking the moral high ground is fine, but few people can easily walk up that mountain to appreciate the view from the other side. Instead, let's take a route all can manage to stop others falling off the cliff. Like teenage dolphins playing with a deadly poison, education and governments should focus on harm reduction rather than simple, ineffective messages of 'no'. You can't remove all the puffer fish from the sea just as you cannot remove all the illicit drugs from the world.

In the two weeks before Kevin jumped from the bridge, he had slept for a total of just two hours. Wrapped in contorted bedclothes like a crumpled tissue, he would wake only to be mocked by his alarm clock, barely minutes having gone by. Lying awake, Kevin swallowed the darkness of the night, making his anxiety worse. He was like a whale but without its purpose.

The 5-tonne orca whale goes without sleep for three months after giving birth to a calf. In today's neon Netflix-impregnated world, many of us are similarly sleep-deprived but without the calf to care for. Humans are the only animal species that purposely goes without sleep when not starving, migrating or trying to escape predators.

Matthew Walker, in his book *Why We Sleep*, argues that unlike other bodily functions, sleep is unique as it lacks a mechanism for storage. Fat cells store calories that can be used long after a feast is over. Unlike batteries that store energy, sleep cannot be banked and used after a late-night welcoming in another New Year. Even small reductions in the quantity or quality of sleep leads to measurable health impacts – higher rates of obesity, cancer, heart disease and depression. Nurses in Denmark won compensation by showing their years of night shifts contributed to the development of their breast cancer. When I retire at the creaking age of sixty-seven, I'll have a lot of night shifts under my belt, loosened to accommodate my shift-work-induced obesity. Catching up on forty-four years of poor sleep needs a very long lie-in and sadly sleeping longer as a catch-up technique doesn't even work. Despite this, society rewards early risers – the early bird is said to catch the worm. But individuals have individual sleep needs and patterns. For some they will never be an early bird, but it's the second mouse that eats the cheese.

Humans are story machines, trying to make sense of the world. Sleep is an essential part of organising, filtering and working through our thoughts. Although Kevin seldom thought about his own sleep before jumping from the Golden Gate Bridge, there is not a single psychiatric condition that has normal sleep patterns. Humans need to listen to our animal ancestors and only deny sleep when hunting, travelling or caring for others. Turn off 'auto-play the next episode' so your life can have another series.

Kevin's bright red jumper flashed on my laptop screen. As the connection stabilised, I could see he was surrounded by superhero comics in his Atlanta home. These are the same comics Kevin had given away the day before he planned to die. Kevin was, and still is, part of a very special 1 per cent; one of just thirty-nine people who survived jumping from the Golden Gate Bridge out of 2,000 others. Almost all of those twenty-six survivors alive today had the same immediate sense of regret as Kevin felt when his hands flung his body over the edge.

His body had slammed against the grey water, shattering his back. The freezing sea temperatures paralysed Kevin's muscles. Unable to swim, his body started sinking. But someone immediately came to the rescue. A brilliant swimmer who could hold their breath for over thirty minutes. Partially conscious, Kevin felt something circling beneath him, holding him afloat on the surface of the water preventing him from downing. Keeping him alive.

'It was Herbert,' Kevin told me. 'A sea lion saved my life.'

Later confirmed by an eyewitness, a sea lion kept Kevin afloat for fifteen minutes before the coastguard arrived. Doctors surgically repaired his body and after four weeks, Kevin started the first of seven in-patient psychiatric stays to deal with depression, paranoia and hallucinations.

Kevin survived thanks to two animals. First, Herbert the sea lion, but then a companion dog, a Shar Pei called Max, who helped him through many of the tough days that followed his survival. Kevin met his future wife, Margaret, while still a psychiatric in-patient by pretending he was a member of staff and finding her telephone number from the hospital's visitor logbook. Margaret wasn't the only human connection Kevin would make. Echoing the animal importance of social connection, he tracked down a long-lost half-sister, half-brother, aunts and cousins from his parents' past. Thanks to this support, Kevin has achieved astonishing things.

In St. Mary's psychiatric hospital, a Franciscan friar named Brother George Cherrie, the hospital's chaplin, encouraged Kevin to tell his story, first to himself and then to millions of others. Seven months after jumping, a hesitant Kevin spoke to 120 schoolchildren with brutal honesty, compassion and living insight about wanting to die. 'I was freaking out,' he says. 'I was a mess.'

Two weeks later, letters arrived from several of the children, telling Kevin to keep talking. To spread his message of hope and honesty. And he did. Kevin now travels the world using his story as a human tool to prevent suicide. His advocacy work led to the film *Suicide: The Ripple Effect*, awarded Best Documentary at BAFTA's Visionary Honours Awards in 2019, with the prize presented to Kevin by Nelson Mandela's grandson. Kevin's adopted father, Patrick Hines, joined Dave Hull and Paul Muller whose lives had also been changed after loved ones had jumped from the Golden Gate Bridge. They formed the Bridge Rail Foundation, helping to erect a physical suicide barrier on the Golden Gate Bridge. This $211 million project, which started in 2018, will use 3.5 miles of netting 20ft below the bridge, extending 20ft out on both sides of the bridge. Due to be completed in 2023, this will hold up people at the brink of crisis even when Herbert the sea lion cannot.

Just as Kevin survived his jump, so too did Hendrix the dog, who leapt from the Scottish bridge. A week after his scraped skin and sprained paw had recovered, Hendrix was back running through the woods near his home. Animal behaviourist David Sands investigated the Dog Suicide Bridge phenomenon and ruled out the possibility that animals were deliberately killing themselves. Instead, his experiments found dogs were drawn to the scent of wildlife below, especially in long-nose breeds like Hendrix. Combined with dogs' limited perspective vision and the bridge path's sudden change in direction, they were enticed to jump.

Kevin's life is still tangled with difficult days, days he hears voices and days he can't leave the house. But sticking to a ten-step plan allows Kevin to keep living rather than trying to die. These steps have loud echoes of the animal lessons from dolphins, whales, monkeys and rats, including prioritising sleep, minimising drug use and ensuring physical connection to others. Kevin thinks of these not as a system of escape, but rather a way to return to human. They are the things that fill the gaps when he feels broken. A bit like the Japanese art of kintsugi – mending broken pottery with melted gold – this is now where life happens, in the in-betweens. Where he met his wife. Where he helps so many others. He has filled these cracks to make a better, new whole.

'When the bad feelings return,' Kevin says, 'I always tell someone who loves me and who cares about me and who empathises with me.

'I have one request of people who are currently facing the struggle, who can't see the light at the end of the tunnel,' he continues. 'Remember the light is there, the hope is there, you have to find a way to make it and find a way to move forward until you reach the hope.'

The last thing he told me, with jaw-tight determination, was: 'I will never die by suicide.'

EPILOGUE

'Clearly, animals know more than we think,
and think a great deal more than we know.'

IRENE M. PEPPERBERG

It was the first time that Mia had diagnosed cancer. She was a specialist in helping people with serious heart conditions, not an oncologist. But she knew there was a problem with Emilie's left breast. She didn't examine Emilie or even ask her any questions. A mammogram or scan wasn't needed. All Mia needed was her nose. She could smell cancer.

Mia wasn't actually a doctor. But she helped Emilie survive each day. When Emilie's serious heart condition caused her to collapse, Mia would call for help and bring the right tablets from Emilie's pocket to help. Smelling Emilie's cancer would also save her life, just as Mia had been saved by Emilie five years earlier from an illegal puppy farm. Because Mia was a miniature dachshund. An assistance dog.

Emilie was training to be a vet when Mia jumped on to her lap and nuzzled the flesh at the top of her left breast. Although trained to help Emilie's deafness and heart condition, Mia closed her eyes and licked furiously, the same way she did to a bruise or cut. They both knew something was wrong. Just a week later, Stage 2 breast cancer was confirmed. After surgery and radiotherapy, Emilie was given the all-clear one year later. She still lives with Mia, caring for many other rescue dogs too, giving them a second chance at life as she had been given.

Although we have long known dogs can smell human disease, this story underlines our two-way relationship with animals. Emilie had helped Mia and Mia helped Emilie. Medicine needs to reimagine its unhappy marriage with animals from one of exploitation to one of reciprocity.

The chain-link fence between human and animal health was prised open long ago. Rudolf Virchow, a prominent nineteenth-century doctor, coined the term 'zoonosis' after finding roundworms in both pigs and humans. He showed how disease could be passed back and forth. I hope this book shows that so can cures.

In the twentieth century, Calvin Schwabe, in his textbook *Veterinary Medicine and Human Health*, coined the term

'One Medicine'. This simple phrase welds together human and veterinary medicine into a whole. And I hope this book shows the urgent need to diagnose, cure, prevent and understand illnesses together, not apart.

In the twenty-first century, Abigail Woods, in her book *Animals and the Shaping of Modern Medicine*, argued that animals have long shaped modern medicine but not benefited from it. Animals have given their lives, for us, with little in return.

Human doctors like me have been peering through this chain-link fence, pressing our faces so close that imprints are left on our faces. The problem is that the fence shouldn't be there at all.

Bringing animals into our circle of concern, into medicine and into our care should not be difficult. Billionaires are looking at other planets to extend humanity into the future. Let's also turn those telescopes towards our Earth, use their power to magnify lives that are not seen or understood. Looking closely will make us realise what we are missing. The greatest living naturalist, David Attenborough, put it starkly when he said: 'We have thought this was our planet. Ninety-six per cent of its mass is us and the animals we eat. We have replaced the wild with the tame. Run for humankind by humankind. We have overrun the Earth.'

Let's use this moment, emerging from the pandemic, to wake up. We have the power to think about and choose the future. It's understandable that many people are in a hurry to return to normal. But I think we should all be in a hurry to remember which parts of normal are really worth returning to. The animals who can help cure cancer, restart a heart, save a brain, stop a pandemic, save a life and save a death are here, under our noses, in our hands, in our homes and under your toes. They live on us and inside us. Humans naturally look to the future and into the distance, but humanity needs to listen to the past, to what is close to us, to what made us.

I grieved when my trip to the faraway Galápagos Islands was stopped by the pandemic. Then I discovered, in the woods where I played as a child, the home of Alfred Russel Wallace. He had written his twenty-two books, 700 articles and co-discovered evolution with Darwin by looking at the animals that I grew up with in my tiny Welsh town of Neath. These answers were found not far away in the Galápagos, but in the river where I threw sticks, in the grass where I lay and in the ground where I had stood. Darwin's closest colleague was under my nose all along. And so are the answers to medicine's trickiest questions. But to find them, we need to change.

This change can start with you. Stop meeting animals as meat, as only items on your plate. Expand your moral circle to include life and not just human life. If you are a doctor, learn from vets. If you train doctors, train with vets. Human doctors swear an oath to just one species while vets include every remaining variety of life. Perhaps they should instead become one. If you train nurses, train with nurses who care for animals. If you are a scientist, learn from animal lives and not just animal deaths. And if you are simply a human, curl yourself around animals when they need you. Remember that the gifts they keep giving us, this sharing between species, carries ethical implications. Working together is for the benefit of all. I now read Darwin's *The Descent of Man* as a book illuminating human connections with the life machinery of animals. The title could instead read 'The Ascent of All' because the sum of these parts are we.

I often stand at that bed space in the intensive care unit where we saved Barry from choking on a biscuit. In his place are other patients with very different problems. Yet there is always an animal to talk about, a species who can help us and who we can help in return. I used to think that I worked only with humans. But now I know I work only with animals.

Acknowledgements

Thanks to all my friends who didn't (out loud) tell me to shut up when talking endlessly about giraffes. A special mention to my good friends who have shared many an evening around a beach fire or at the Sully Inn. Thanks to Barney for telling me about the Golden Gate Bridge, to Cai for asking me to speak, to Jake for his wonderful photos. Thanks to Lowri and Laura for reading early versions of this book. Thanks to Between The Trees for a platform to think about this book. Thanks to my parents and family who have supported trips away, Sundays in coffee shops and evenings typing away with Joni Mitchell on loop and incense burning.

It is thanks to the wonderful Charlotte Seymour at Johnson & Alcock that my words have found these pages at all, along with brilliant guidance from Frances Jessop and Fritha Saunders at Simon & Schuster and the team at Andrew Nurnberg. Thanks to David Edwards who helped make this book much better.

Thanks to Dafydd Parry and Gary Thomas who

encouraged my early interest in animal physiology rather than revising for exams. Hugh Montgomery told me some remarkable things about animals that are included in this book. Thanks to Peter, Tracey and Moose Brindley (as well as the bees) who gave me their home and their welcome. Richard Anderson told me the amazing story about the whale's heart and Scott Bradburn introduced me to some great authors. Luke Lewis from the late STA Travel helped organise my trips and Robert Macfarlane helped inspire my choice of words.

Thanks to Jade and Stuart for their insights about our therapy dog. Thanks to Justine Shotton and the BVA, Tracey King and the Humanimal Trust, and Noel Fitzpatrick and his team. Sarah Carter and Richard Huxtable helped find my old dissertation that I thought was long shredded. Pippa Hardman with Natural Resources Wales, the South Wales Caving Club and George Nash worked hard to organise the rock art visit that has such an impact on this book. Thanks to Andrew and Dawn from Between the Trees and Sophia Salmon.

To my wonderful colleagues at the University Hospital of Wales, BMJ, the Royal Perth Hospital, WACHS, Curtin University and Cardiff University – thank you for your hard work, support and care. You make work feel less like work and more like time spent with friends. It has been a tough few years that we will not forget.

Thanks to Paul Craddock, Paul Ponganis, Michael Jaeger, Jono Lineen, Ilora Finlay, Dean Burnett, Chris Baraniuk, Jane Common, Hein Wellens, Sylvia van der Straten,

Acknowledgements

Roberto Kolter, Lyndy Cooke, Ulyseese (the Software) and the people on Ellen Shona.

But most of all, thank you to the scientists, the patients, their friends, their families, the people and the animals who have spoken to me and I have written about. I hope I have done your stories justice, especially those who cannot read what I have written.

INDEX

Index

Index

Index